Systemic Constellations

Systemic Constellations

Theory, Practice, and Applications

Damian Janus

Translated by Barbara Gąstoł

LEXINGTON BOOKS

Lanham • Boulder • New York • London

Published by Lexington Books
An imprint of The Rowman & Littlefield Publishing Group, Inc.
4501 Forbes Boulevard, Suite 200, Lanham, Maryland 20706
www.rowman.com

6 Tinworth Street, London SE11 5AL, United Kingdom

British Library Cataloguing in Publication Information Available

Library of Congress Cataloging-in-Publication Data

Names: Janus, Damian, 1969- author. | Gąstoł, Barbara, translator.
Title: Systemic constellations : theory, practice, and applications / Damian Janus ; translated by, Barbara Gąstoł.
Other titles: Ustawienia systemowe Berta Hellingera. English.
Description: Lanham : Lexington Books, [2021] | Translation of: Ustawienia systemowe Berta Hellingera : przełom w psychoterapii i wiedzy o człowieku. | Includes bibliographical references and index.
Identifiers: LCCN 2021003090 (print) | LCCN 2021003091 (ebook) | ISBN 9781793627452 (cloth) | ISBN 9781793627469 (ebook)
Subjects: LCSH: Hellinger, Bert. | Systemic therapy (Family therapy) | Family constellations (Families)
Classification: LCC RC488.5 .J352 2021 (print) | LCC RC488.5 (ebook) | DDC 616.89/156—dc23
LC record available at https://lccn.loc.gov/2021003090
LC ebook record available at https://lccn.loc.gov/2021003091

Contents

Introduction

Systemic constellations that are the subject of this book are a breakthrough method of psychotherapy, coaching, and consulting. The potential of the approach developed by Bert Hellinger significantly surpasses the capabilities of most traditional psychotherapeutic and counseling methods. Systemic constellations can be used with equal success to improve mental functioning, better interpersonal relationships, help overcome health problems and life difficulties, and achieve specific life or professional goals. They can be used to help both adults and small children, and their effects, according to numberless accounts of clients, are sometimes completely transformative.

How is it possible that the same method can be used both to solve psychophysical problems of an infant and to deal with financial difficulties in a company? It transpires that similar systemic processes determine the functioning of all human systems—family, cohabiting, professional, and organizational ones. These processes, although extremely important, were so far largely unnoticed, and the causes of the difficulties were attributed to other factors which are in fact not decisive. Thanks to Hellinger's work and systemic constellations, we have discovered these new territories that cause our life, professional, and health problems, but we have also received new tools to deal with these problems.

Systemic constellations are based on a very simple technique that has become the key to discovering hidden relationships. It consists in asking any persons, for example, workshop group participants, to "be" the client's family members (or to represent, for example, the company and its customers where business issues are involved). We do not suggest anything to these persons, we do not expect them to particularly "feel themselves into" their roles or to play a given scenario. This—probably the simplest possible—procedure yields unexpected results. The representatives feel that they want to behave in this manner and not differently, that they want to approach one of the persons, and that they start to be afraid of somebody else or feel angry with them. In this way, the workshop participants bring to light the deep truth about a given system, about the attitudes, dependencies, emotions, and even certain events that probably took place within the family or company.

In the book—divided into two parts—I describe most aspects of the systemic constellation method, also referred to as family constellations. In the first part, I present the theory and analyze the therapist's work and the course of the therapeutic process; I also describe the phenomena characteristic of this method and feelings of the participants. In the second part, I address various application areas of systemic constellations, such as mental and physical health, relationships, work, and business. In this section, I cite many examples of therapy sessions.

Part I

THEORY, PRACTICE, PHENOMENOLOGY

Chapter 1

Systemic Constellations—Fundamentals of the Method

THE THEORY OF SYSTEMIC CONSTELLATIONS

Systemic Constellations—What Is That?

The systemic constellation method was born from the rediscovery of what has long been referred to as the "family system." The author of systemic constellations, Bert Hellinger, deepened and clarified previous observations and conclusions and identified new laws governing family systems. He showed that the impact of one's family is greater than previously assumed. The family system goes far beyond those who interact directly; it includes not only the living but also the dead, and sometimes also nonrelatives. What is most important in the family and has the strongest influence on its members has usually little to do with what happens in the family on the overt level, for example, who we spend time with and who we are consciously attached to within the family. The essence of the system is primarily the unconscious and hidden connections. They are not formed incidentally, when the family members enter into direct relations, but persist regardless of their mutual behaviors, emotions, attitudes, or ideas. We cannot leave the family system or replace it with another one. It does not matter whether we keep in contact with the family members or live alone, whether we are young or at the end of our lives—the family stays with us and affects our fate.[1]

The discovery of these facts became possible due to the unusual phenomenon that can be called the effect of representation. It consists in the fact that if someone asks another person to "be" for a moment, say, his father, then such a procedure will show the essence of his real relationship with his father. It is enough for the other person to "follow his movement," that is, to behave spontaneously and let the impulses that appear in himself direct him. It can be said that this phenomenon is the simplest imaginable psychological technique—there is no instruction here except "Follow your movement," which basically amounts to the tautology: "Do what you will do." Perhaps the phenomenon remained unnoticed for so long because of this extreme simplicity. It is the core of constellations, enabling one to discover the pictures of hidden relations and dynamics in the family system. The information obtained in this way is not only nonrandom, but refers to the issues that are crucial for our health and well-being. This information always shows the client's life and family, not the internal states or personal situation of the representatives who "enact" the system members.[2] These data are so detailed that they reveal concealed adoptions, mental disorders of grandparents, or the existence of half-siblings.

The phenomenon of revealing facts, and not own fantasies, by role-players was observed earlier, but the systemic laws were only identified by Bert Hellinger. Working with representatives made it possible for him to discover the dynamics governing family systems, as well as the influence of the family on the individual. Regardless of whether the constellations took place in Germany or in Japan, characteristic feelings and reactions of the representatives were the same. The actions suggested to the representatives, such as bowing, lying down on the floor, stepping backward or forward, and simple sentences such as "Thank you" or "I leave what's yours with you," always produced the same results. These patterns were distinguished and collectively defined by Hellinger as the orders of love (German *Ordnungen der Liebe*).

Using constellations enables the client and his family system to reenter the path of these orders. Although they are unconsciously desired by us, in real life we sometimes transgress them. This creates a disorder and transgenerational negative interaction between the family members. Are these influences of the family system substantial? Observations made by constellation facilitators, as well as clients' numerous accounts leave no doubt that these are factors of great strength. The influence of the disordered family system along with the client's unconscious attitude is the cause of many negative phenomena: from life failures and bad mood, through mental problems and professional difficulties, to serious illnesses, accidents, and suicides. This does not mean, of course, that the family is the source of problems. On the contrary, bringing about the systemic orders makes it possible to leave what burdened us and to open ourselves to the strength that flows from our ancestors, and thus to regain health, ability to cope with life and well-being.

General Picture of a Constellation

There are various forms of constellations: group, individual, so-called "classic," or silent. Below, I present the most illustrative form—a classic group constellation.

Before the actual constellation, during the initial interview, the therapist asks the client about the problem and basic facts of his life, he asks about his parents and grandparents, he asks if the client has any siblings, whether some family members died prematurely, whether there was a child who died or was aborted, if someone was excluded from the family or experienced a particularly difficult plight. The therapist can also ask about potential perinatal complications, and whether the client was separated from the parents in early childhood. Then, he asks the client to choose a representative of himself and representatives of his family members from among the people present. If this is the first constellation of a given client, we usually ask him to choose representatives of his mother, father, siblings, and sometimes grandparents. The client touches the representatives, saying: "You are me," "You are my father," and so forth. In this way, the respective "roles" are assigned.

In the original version of constellations, the client's task was also to position the representatives in a manner that corresponded to his "inner image of his family" (which usually amounted to spontaneous positioning). This element is currently omitted—it is enough to select a representative and let him stand anywhere in the workshop room. The client can also not put his hands on the representative's shoulders and just ask him to—as we call it—enter the field, that is, to get up from the chair and stand as this or that person. The process will take place anyway. It also happens that the therapist does not even expect a clear definition of the problem, assuming that what is important for the client will be revealed by the constellation anyway. The initial interview can be reduced to presenting the problem. It is also not necessary that the client chooses all the representatives, this can be done by the therapist (at workshops conducted by Hellinger, he usually chose them from the people who raised their hands).

Generally speaking, a constellation consists of two pictures and is a process of moving from the first picture—containing information about the root of problems, to the second picture—indicating and causing the solution. When the constellation starts, the representatives usually immediately begin to have feelings specific to a given constellation. They experience a variety of sensations in their bodies, adopt specific attitudes, and feel particular emotions toward other "family members," their mood changes. The most significant reaction is movement—approaching or moving away from the others, a need to lie down on the floor, walking back and forth, or stiffening. Representatives' sensations are very strong and have nothing to do with their previous state. Representatives may even experience symptoms characteristic of the diseases that the represented people suffer from, they may have heart palpitations or a heartache, nausea, feel pain in their arms or legs, numbness or heat in some part of their bodies. These symptoms—although evident—are not permanent or dangerous, because they disappear when the orders of love are brought about and the constellation ends.

The therapist, continuing the diagnostic process, sometimes brings in additional representatives, for example, grandparents, or changes their mutual positions. He does the latter according to some general resolution patterns, such as setting up the representatives of children in front of the parents, or the siblings in one line. After every such intervention, he asks the representatives how they feel now ("How's that?," "What does the mother feel?," "Has anything changed now?," "Is it better or worse?"). Their feelings indicate what the next step in the constellation should be. The picture of resolution emerges spontaneously, although the therapist, guided by the systemic laws (the orders of love), can facilitate this. He suggests a certain spatial arrangement, proposes certain sentences (so-called "sentences of strength"), or brings in additional representatives.

At the end, the client himself is brought in the constellation, he stands next to his representative or in his place. In this way, he is confronted with the picture of resolution from the inside. The constellation ends when both the representatives and the client—having taken appropriate places and uttered certain words—feel a significant psychophysical relief. It is a sure indicator that the orders of love have been brought about. This final constellation—along with the process that led to it—has an impact both on the client's present condition and on his future life, as it translates into the order in the real family system.

The orders that the therapist brings about are not arbitrary. In principle, they are discovered by the representatives. This happens during almost every constellation and is especially evident during so-called "silent constellations," in which the whole process takes place almost without the therapist's intervention. I mentioned before that a constellation consists of two pictures: a diagnostic picture and a picture of resolution. This is a simplification, as during the session, we move to the resolution pattern smoothly. Constellations show clear teleology—they spontaneously develop from the initial moment, that indicates problems in the system, to the moment the conflict situations are resolved and reconciliation is possible.

When the picture of resolution cannot be fully reached, for example, due to the client's difficulty in accepting the change, the constellation is sometimes interrupted at the point at which the problem is signalized. Such a constellation is also of therapeutic value, because the client is confronted with the structure of the system and his resistance, which increases his awareness and understanding of the problem. However, usually, with the right amount of patience, we manage to reach the picture of resolution.

The Knowing Field

As I said, Bert Hellinger's therapeutic technique is based on the representation of members of the client's family system by strangers and the spontaneous discovery of the actual dependencies within the system. Representatives do not play imposed roles, neither are they guided by their own projections. They build a picture of relations within the family system thanks to the intention to represent other people, through spontaneous movement, and the feelings that arise in them (e.g., an attraction or an antipathy). Usually, the client very quickly notices that the constellation concerns his family and that the representatives show significant similarities to its members. What is important—the constellation reveals also the hidden aspects of the family relationships. They may be surprising in the beginning, but the clients always reach the point where they feel that these unconscious elements are also part of their family reality and their psyche.

How is it possible that in such a simple way we acquire the knowledge that is not available to ordinary perception? The exact mechanism of this phenomenon is unknown. Its hypothetical basis has been referred to as the knowing field (German *wissende Feld*). Although we do not know the nature of this field, the term itself seems adequate. In constellations, the knowing field manifests itself in the form of feelings, impulses, and, above all, movements that come from within the representatives. Sometimes, some words or longer thoughts come to their minds. These elements relate to the actual relations present in the client's system, which can be checked by confronting the results of the constellation with the factual data concerning a given family. The representatives' feelings are often very strong and surprising (the need to bow, body trembling, sadness, pain in some part of the body, anger, weakness in the legs, etc.).

The nature of the knowing field manifests itself also in situations where someone from the group of observers feels that they must enter the constellation, as if they were captivated by some external force. It usually turns out that they start to represent a person who is important for the system and was absent in the constellation before.

The information we obtain through the knowing field is independent of the representative's judgments, attitudes, or knowledge. For example, during a group workshop, a client talks about her grandfather, expresses her grudge against him, complaints about his bad behavior, his tyrannizing her and the family, and does not spare the dramatic details. After she describes him, one of the participants, who, after all, listened to what she said, and certainly did not approve of that behavior, is set up as the grandfather, and another participant is set up as the granddaughter. There is no sign of aggression or tyranny, instead, the grandfather shows affection for the granddaughter, and there is a completely different dynamics that leads him. The representative's previous knowledge and attitude did not disturb the constellation process.

We are used to the vision of the psyche as extremely susceptible to suggestion or driven primarily by what results from its own history. Systemic constellations show the opposite phenomenon—man's ability to experience the states that do not depend on his attitude or knowledge. We assume that the knowing field is the basis of this phenomenon, because it is thanks to it that there are processes that lead to this information.

Factors Shaping Relationships and the System Dynamics

Bert Hellinger identified four basic factors that shape interpersonal relationships and the dynamics of family systems. These are the right to belong, bond, system hierarchy, and the principle of balance. Systemic constellations enable a diagnosis of disturbances within these four dynamics and bring the orders of love into the system, which leads to balance in the system and well-being and development of its members.

Hellinger discovered the orders of love by observing repetitive feelings and behaviors of representatives. These behaviors—such as spontaneous bowing down before the parents—bring relief to the client's representative (remember that he is neutral toward the client's problem) and have a positive impact on the other representatives. They emerge spontaneously in many different constellations, without being in any way Hellinger's creation. If we collect such spontaneous "interventions" of representatives from a few dozens of constellations, we will have a full catalog of systemic orders.

Essentially, the orders of love consist in bringing the excluded ones back in the family system (e.g., the aborted child who was not considered a family member); bringing the bonds between the members of the family system to light (e.g., with the previously unknown biological father); restoring the hierarchy that plays an important role in the family (e.g., between the parents and children); giving back or accepting one's own responsibility (e.g., no longer taking on the parent's problems); proper balancing (e.g., by thanking the adoptive parents internally); and accepting masculine or feminine identification by mental "standing side by side" with the father or mother.

The orders of love are universal and apply to all people regardless of their history, personality, or attitude. Bringing about these orders in a constellation always results in relief, a sense of unburdening (a characteristic psychophysical feeling of getting rid of the "load"), and new energy. Sometimes there is a need for an exception to one of the orders, but this is very rare. For instance, in a situation where the mother is particularly heavily systemically burdened or moves toward death, despite the fact that generally the daughter should "stand by the mother" (and the son by the father), in this case, the daughter must "stand by the father." This means that she can only identify herself to a minimal extent with what comes from the mother. However, there is no exception to the more basic orders, such as the need to maintain the hierarchy between the parents and children.

The orders of love also include accepting the parents; honoring the previous partner so that a new relationship can succeed; leaving the child who lost his parents in his biological family (if possible); in the case of adoption—honoring the biological parents; in the case of divorce—honoring the other parent in the child; counting the stillborn baby with the other siblings; respect for the bond that arises between the victim and the perpetrator in the case of sexual abuse.

Belonging

The right to belong is the most basic system dynamics. No one can be excluded from the system with impunity. Everyone who has ever belonged has the right to still belong. The system "remembers" all its elements. When someone is excluded, the other system members will suffer consequences. What does exclusion consist in? It is forgetting someone, ignoring them, negating their meaning, concealing their existence, or demonizing them. It may also be idealizing someone, putting them on the pedestal. In this way, a given person is divested of the status of an ordinary man and a family member, and in this case, one cannot fully accept them. I remember a situation where the client's grandfather, a patriot, a veteran of the World War I and victim of the World War II, was excluded in some sense, because his heroism and the memory of his death was in the foreground. Neither the son nor the grandson (the client) could regard him simply as a father and grandfather. This state of affairs blocked the flow of energy, which was also reflected in the attitude of the client's son (the great-grandson).

Exclusion also arises when someone has not reconciled himself to someone else's death. For example, when the mother cannot accept her first child's death, the family does not talk about him and he, as it were, ceases to exist. By not accepting that the child has died, the family negates the child's existence, both past and present—in the spiritual form, in the memory of its members. They do not think of him as one of the siblings. And they do not give him a place in the family system.

Exclusion takes place very often. The excluded include divorced fathers, alcoholic parents, half-siblings, children who died early or were aborted, the mentally ill and handicapped, ex-partners, people whose lot was so traumatic that the others do not want to remember it, killers, as well as victims of homicides and accidents if their deaths were caused by someone in our family. Exclusions do not have to be "malicious"—as it often happens in the case of negating the importance of a child's father or mother—paradoxically, they may result from pain and bereavement. In this way, children who died shortly after birth may be excluded. Their death is such a great trauma for their parents that they are unable to think about it and do not want to remember it. They may want to have another child to, as it were, erase the horrible memory of the deceased one.

Each exclusion greatly destabilizes the entire system. We can refer here in part to the theory of systems—any system devoid of one of the elements seeks to maintain the *status quo*. For this purpose, another element must take over the functions of the excluded element. In Hellinger's theory, we call this entanglement. It consists in the fact that one of the family members unconsciously identifies with the excluded person. In this way, he includes that person back in the system.

The Bond

There is a bond between all members of the family. The strongest bond is the one between children and parents, between siblings and those whose lot was a hard one. There is also a bond between a woman and a man in an intense sexual relationship. It is particularly strong when the woman became pregnant, even if the child was not born, and the partners did not consciously care about each other. A certain type of bond forms even as a result of rape or sexual abuse in childhood.

What is a bond? It is a kind of primal love and it is unwitting, unaffected by one's personal assessments, or consciously experienced feelings toward a given person. One can hate their mother or father and the bond with them remains anyway. It is also a kind of unconscious reaction and unconscious knowledge about other members of the system. As a result of the existence of the bond, what happens to one member of the family is not immaterial to the others. The bond is a form of fidelity, which is observed most of all in children who are attached to their parents regardless of who they are and how they act toward them. The bond is followed by primal loyalty. That is why children want to share the lot of their parents and family regardless of what it is. When there is something on the conscious level that some people describe as a lack of bond, nothing changes on the primal level, and the unconscious bond with the parents and other family members remains forever.

The bond affects our lives and connects our fate with the fate of the other family members. Although we remain unaware of its strength, the bond manifests in many conscious ways. Someone may feel as if they were attached to another person, although they have no idea who the other person is. This is the case for adopted children, separated siblings, and twins. One man, who found his twin brother after nearly 70 years, said, "I've always felt that I have a brother somewhere. And I said so to my friends."

This unconscious bond is an extremely important factor shaping our lives. If we are attached to the people we have never been aware of, we struggle—we try to understand ourselves, our partners, and cope with children, but do not succeed. This is the fate of many adopted people who were not told about the adoption. They may repetitively dream about the people who seem important to them, but they cannot recognize them. When they finally find out about their adoption, when they find the names of their mother, father, and siblings, then their bond becomes conscious, which brings them peace. One of such persons said:

> The fact that I found my roots and met my sister changed my life. I had never been able to find myself. I had been constantly changing jobs and partners. I had submitted to my [adoptive] mother, then to men. I had never known what I had wanted. When I met Alice [sister], everything started to fall into place. I have a permanent job, I have built a new relationship and there is someone I can ask for help. We talk with Alice openly, I seek her advice when I have a problem with something. She supports me. I have stopped being unquiet, since I won her back. (Kamińska 2016, 5)[3]

Hierarchy

In the system, there is a hierarchy that consists in a one-way flow from the older (the earlier ones in the system) to the younger (the later ones). The older ones give (it flows through them), and the younger ones take (it comes to them). The hierarchy is something that physicists refer to as the "arrow of time." It determines the direction of the flow, of both good and bad things, of burdens and traumas, but also strength and energy. We say that the older take precedence over the younger: older siblings take precedence over the younger ones, and parents over children. What does this mean exactly? The place of the earlier cannot be taken or underestimated by those who joined later. The latter must accept that they are heirs, not creators. They must agree that something comes to them and that they cannot give back against the current. What comes from parents to children, and never the other way around? Above all, the gift of life. It may seem obvious, but some people would like to pay back to their parents for life (sometimes probably because they think they would not have to be eternally grateful this way). This attitude is like trying to turn back the river. The one who violates the hierarchy seems to oppose the course of time, the fact that first there were older ones and then there came younger ones. He weakens instead of drawing strength.

The hierarchy can also be violated by parents. Sometimes someone says that they "learn from their children" or that he is their "friend." Of course, this may happen, and it may be good. However, at a deeper level, there is no two-way interchange between parents and children. Parents are always donors, children are recipients, and it is not possible to change this order. When it is difficult for the parent to recognize this law and he puts the child on the same level or above himself, he always burdens the child. The hierarchy between parents and children is a basic one, but the hierarchical order applies to everyone in the family. The hierarchy between siblings is also important. An older brother shapes us much stronger than a younger one, regardless of the real contact with them. Older siblings are more important to our lives than younger ones, regardless of the feelings we have for them.

Balance

The balancing mechanism means that we automatically try to balance what is given with what is taken. And it also applies to what we do to others and what we experienced from them. If we receive, we have a reflex to repay. If we hurt someone, there is a desire to hurt ourselves too, or to be punished. If, in turn, someone hurts us and we suffer, we want to take revenge on them so that they also suffer. It is as if we were keeping internal accounts, trying to balance "revenues" with "expenses."

The balance of giving and taking has a profound influence on our frame of mind. The one who gives, feels free, entitled to demands, better. The one who takes is burdened with guilt, feels obliged and worse. When I pay back to the other as much as I received, I unburden myself of my obligations and feel free. When I pay back more, I believe I am entitled to something and I experience it as a specific kind of innocence. When I cannot repay, I feel enslaved, obliged, and guilty. If one of the partners only gives and the other cannot pay back, then the latter will show a tendency to end the relationship. Why? He will not be able to bear his own sense of obligation and inferiority. It will be so even when on a conscious level he only wants to take and does not think about giving anything in return, for the balancing mechanism works under the threshold of consciousness.

The balance between give and take works out well for relationships—of both good and bad things. For example, when someone does not demand reparation from the perpetrator and says hastily that he "forgives" him, it is not in favor of the relationship. The perpetrator, unable to satisfy the need for balance and take an equal position, must leave. The relationship can only last if there is no significant disproportion in receiving and giving. As Hellinger says, the relationship develops if one repays for good with a bit more good, and for evil—with a little less evil. It ends when there is complete balance or when one of the partners refuses to give or take.

There is yet another process that can also be described as balancing. While the process referred to above is automatic and unconscious, this one can only be done intentionally, generally during a constellation. It is giving back "what is not mine" or taking "what is mine." As children, we tend to take on ourselves anything that burdens our parents. Thanks to the unconscious perception, we know about their loads, guilt, pain, depression, and try to relieve them. We imagine that we can bear their difficulties. It will be balancing to give back to the parents what is their concern and what the child has taken unconsciously on himself. There is also another side to it. Although we unconsciously shoulder other people's baggage, we often turn away from our own loads. For example, we do not want to admit our own guilt. When those to whom the guilt belongs admit it, and those who carry the guilt that is not theirs give it back, then this kind of balancing takes place. It is a psycho-physical sensation, as if a physical burden were involved. When the client's representative says that he "leaves what is not his," he feels relieved, and so does the client himself.

Boundaries of the Family System

The boundaries of the family system are defined quite precisely. The following people always belong to each person's system:

- His parents and their siblings (also half-siblings, deceased, stillborn, and aborted ones);
- Siblings (half-siblings, deceased, stillborn, and aborted ones);
- Grandparents, sometimes some of their siblings (this happens rarely);
- Often great-grandparents;
- Those who made room in the system for others (ex-wives and ex-husbands, ex-fiancés and ex-fiancées, ex-partners);
- Those who acted in the interest of the system, and who suffered great harm, also those at whose expense someone in the system benefited significantly (e.g., disinherited persons);
- Killers and their victims;
- Sometimes participants in brutal war events.

What exactly does it mean that these people belong to the system? It means that they have an impact on a given person. Note that these are basically the "earlier," older than him (the exception is siblings, who may be younger, but have an impact on the individual because of the strength of the mutual bond, although, experience has shown that older siblings have a stronger impact). The family system normally consists of related people, but unrelated people can also enter it. They usually are parents' former partners. Not necessarily all former partners; however, the persons who always belong to the system are the ones that were harmed, abandoned, or when there was a pregnancy in the relationship.

The fact that not only relatives belong to the system is Bert Hellinger's significant discovery. Consider a therapeutic example. Margaret[4] lived in her childhood with her father, mother, and his former wife, Lucy, which she considered to be a very strange situation that negatively affected her life. Later Lucy moved to residential care, and Margaret remained with her parents in the apartment. In the constellation, the representative of Lucy just wanted only to be seen and acknowledged. It turned out that the ex-wife, if internally accepted by the client, could become a source of strength for her. Margaret perceived her as just a ball and chain in her childhood. Now it turned out that in her inner world she had assumed the role of almost a second mother. Why was she so important? As her father's previous partner, she was the one who sacrificed a lot for Margaret's family. This is how it looks from the point of view of the family conscience. That is why she entered her system. When Margaret's representative hugged Lucy's representative, the client clearly felt that something was completed. The pain caused by the "abnormal" situation of her childhood disappeared. Thanks to Lucy, Margaret had more, not less, as she had thought before.

In another constellation, a complete stranger turned out to matter. During Josephine's constellation one of the workshop participants felt that she should enter its field (which happens in constellations with experienced representatives). When the person entered, the client said that as an infant she was hospitalized because of pneumonia. She probably got sick because of the nurse's mistake. It became clear that the unidentified person was probably that nurse (oddly enough her representative was dressed in a simple blue dress, resembling a nurse's outfit). What was important here? It was crucial for the client to accept that person as the cause of her own fate, in particular to accept the fact that the bond with her mother was interrupted because of the nurse's mistake—to accept without reproach and without underestimating its meaning. As can be seen in the last two examples, what brings a person into the system (makes him important for the client's psychic life) is the strength of his impact on the most significant aspects of life at an early stage. In the case of Margaret, it was a person who had to "lose" for Margaret to be born, and in the case of Josephine, it was a person whose conduct greatly influenced her whole life.

Victims and killers also belong to the system. Not only perpetrators of murders, as some accidents have the same effect. The constellation of Abigail, whose father died in a car accident, seemed to be at a standstill. I could not bring this constellation to an end, as the representatives were restless. I intuitively asked how the father had died. It turned out that he had been changing a wheel and got hit by another driver. Only after bringing in the representative of that driver the system calmed down and the constellation could be completed. The driver was actually the killer of the client's father, he was connected with this system and was important here.

As I mentioned before, the system also includes deceased and aborted children. Miscarriages—as my experience shows—usually do not belong to the system.[5] A natural miscarriage may be a psychologically difficult situation for the mother, but it has no systemic significance, meaning it is unlikely to burden younger siblings. However, if the child is already so developed that he could potentially live independently, then we deal with a death rather than a miscarriage, and this has a systemic meaning. It is different in the case of abortion—it seems that abortion at every stage of fetal life entails the existence of the child in the system. As if the act of abortion constitutes him as a human being.

A very important person in the system, whose influence may be noticeable over many generations, is a woman who died in childbirth. The influence of this event may be manifested in the female line of the family, for example, in the form of difficulty in accepting the role of a mother, fear of childbirth, and problems with procreation. I facilitated a constellation where such a death probably happened six to seven generations earlier and continued to affect the following ones. When it comes to men, Hellinger argues that some suicide acts are an attempt to pay for the death of a woman in childbirth. This is because in the family system there appears an unconscious conviction that it was a man who contributed to the death of the woman through sex.

The Systemic Role of the Deceased

One of Hellinger's most important findings is that in the family system an important role is played not only by the living but also by the deceased. The individual is influenced by both those he contacts on a daily basis and by the other members of his family, regardless of whether they live or not. Hellinger argues that

> In keeping with what we experience and the effects we can observe, it would seem as if the dead remain with us for a while. They are gone in that we can't see them any longer, but they are still present through their effects on us, as if they were still there. (Hellinger 2003, 112)

> All those who can be remembered, back to the grandparents' generation—sometimes as far back as the great-grandparents—have an effect as if they were there. (Hellinger and Hövel 1999, 57)

> The dead who are not honored or grieved for, or who are simply forgotten, seem to stay around an especially long time. (Hellinger 2003, 127)

The dead are not just memories. When we position the deceased parents, we will see their mutual relations, the character of which will not depend on our memories (similarly, the roles of the living are not built from what we know about them). We will see how difficult it is for our mother to accept her own mother, even though they are both dead. We will see the dynamics of the deceased who had passed away before we were born, including those whose existence we have never been aware of. The dead do not disappear from the system, but they exist through their influence. The effects of transgressing the orders of love—such as exclusion, rejection of the parent, breaking the hierarchy, not taking the blame, and so on—by the deceased do not disappear from the system either. If the deceased mother did not take responsibility for her abortion, her living child may take it on himself. If she did not accept her mother, her daughter may find it harder to accept her as a mother. Victims of homicides and killers, children that died early, or parents who died when their children were small, have a particularly strong effect. Their exclusion may be the cause of many problems and diseases, and including them again in the system makes their impact either positive or weaker.

Hellinger says that not only the dead affect the living, the living can also affect the dead. What does it mean? This happens during a constellation in which the dead are honored by the fact that they are included in the system. The beneficial effects of such an act are manifested through the representatives' feelings. The representative of the dead calms down, closes his eyes and, as it were, tunes out the constellation. Also, the other representatives who were anxious calm down, and the ones who were deprived of their strength—feel an inflow of energy. Because we can see here the interdependence of the living and the dead, we can say that we "do something for the deceased."

All in all, however, a constellation always serves the living and life and—of course—it has nothing to do with spiritualism. The fact that the dead made "alive" by representatives acquire a kind of existence and autonomy, enables the client to go much further than it would be possible if we worked only with his memories. If someone did not reconcile with his parents, holds a grudge or feels angry with one of them, he can change it during a constellation. It will be the same work as the one he would do if his parents were alive.

One should bear in mind that constellations reveal first of all the orders of love, someone's difficult plight, and the character of a given relationship, for example, whether the parents were strongly attached or rather distanced themselves from each other. During constellations, we will not find out where the great-grandfather buried his coins or what political views he shared. The dead can be a source of disharmony or support a given person, but it does not mean that some of them are "mean" and others "kind." It is primarily a matter of the (unconscious) attitude of the living person toward them. Someone may consider a deceased person a threat or follow him into death, but the movement springs just from themselves, not from the character of the deceased.

Primary and Secondary Feelings

Some of our affects are not essential and are secondary to much more important primary emotions. Nevertheless, many therapeutic methods focus on these secondary emotions, assuming that they are the cause or an essential element of human problems. The emotion, which is often demonized and whose importance is overestimated, is anger. Constellations show that anger or aggression are not primary and often mask something completely different. Hellinger maintains that anger often replaces sadness, it is used to defend against guilt, and it may also be a substitute for action. I can be angry because I notice that I did not take something I could or should have taken; I can be angry instead of showing love (which I cannot do because of the interrupted movement of love); I can be angry with someone because I have wronged him, or because I cannot repay someone who gives me a lot. There may also be anger that is absolutely not mine, which is taken over from someone else (Hellinger 2001, 167–69).

Aggressive behaviors have their roots, and saying that someone is aggressive because "that is their character" or "they were born like this" is incorrect. When a representative in a constellation feels angry, wants to impose something or arouses fear, it usually means that there is still something missing in the constellation, something that is the cause of this behavior. When we bring in a representative of "aggression" or its cause, his behavior will change, his aggression will disappear, and may be replaced by a picture of bond. It turns out in such cases that aggression was only a reaction to a disorder in the system or a trauma. This is what mattered from the systemic point of view and had a negative effect on the client and other people in the family. So the source of the problems is not, for example, the person's bad temper, because the bad temper itself was a reaction to something more fundamental, often to exclusion.

When we look at family systems and the functioning of individual people, it turns out that behind the most destructive behaviors there is the original bond. Everyone is submerged in it, and those who seem to be the worst, are sometimes particularly attached and loyal. Would it make sense to dwell on anger, grievance, animosity, or humiliation? From the systemic point of view, these are secondary emotions that, at most, indicate something much more basic.

Another example of the impact of primary feelings is sexual abuse. It generates shame, fear, and anger in the victim. These unpleasant emotions are often reinforced by the reactions of the relatives, friends, or therapists. In some cases, excessive excitation, "falling in love" with the perpetrator, or compulsive sexual behavior may occur. In constellations, we discover that these emotions are secondary, triggered by something that lies deeper. This something is the involuntary bond that formed between the victim and the perpetrator. It will have a particularly strong impact on the victim's life. Realizing this and expressing the automatically formed bond invariably brings relief and liberation.

Of course, secondary emotions are normal and impossible to avoid. However, discovering primary feelings gives strength and is the goal of therapy.

CAUSES OF LIFE PROBLEMS, MENTAL DISORDERS, AND SOMATIC DISEASES

Systemic Determinants of Disorders

Systemic constellations shed new light on the issue of development and persistence of the most serious diseases and disorders, both mental and somatic, as well as life and professional difficulties. It turned out that these—so diverse—phenomena may have similar systemic causes, because systemic disorder can manifest itself in the relational or professional sphere as well as in the psychic and physical sphere.

Hellinger presented his observations on disorders and illnesses in the form of simple patterns. He said that

- Anorexia is saying to the parent: "I'll disappear in your place, dear dad," and also sympathizing with the excluded or withdrawn father;
- Anorexia of the bulimic type is the oscillation between the attitude of "I live" and "I disappear";
- Bulimia is the ability to take only from the mother, but sympathizing with the father by spitting out what was taken from the mother;
- Compulsive overeating in women is eating the excluded "part" of the mother;
- Neurosis is the interrupted movement of love;
- Psychosis results from the identification with the victim and the perpetrator of a murder, identification with a person of the opposite sex, self-punishment for assuming the role of the parent's partner;
- Schizophrenia is a murder within the family;
- Autism is the withdrawal as a defense against murderous impulses caused by identification with the murderer;

- Depression occurs when one or both parents have been rejected or when access to one of them was impossible;
- Manic-depressive psychosis is the sexualization of the parent-child relationship, incest (as observed by Franz Ruppert);
- Mania is identification with someone who is dead, who is "in heaven";
- Speech disorders (stuttering) take place when one of the family members could not be heard, two persons in the family were conflicted with each other (e.g., as a victim and perpetrator), when there is identification with someone who arouses fear;
- Addiction is the search for the father, who could not be accessed because of the mother, at the same time it is taking revenge on the mother;
- Heavy addiction, such as heroinism, is a hidden attempt of suicide, saying: "I'll follow you," "Rather me than you," or "I'll die with you";
- Cancer is "incomplete bowing down," atonement for one's own or adopted guilt (abortion, giving a child away), following someone into death, excessive giving, and inability to take from the mother;
- Multiple sclerosis means: "I'll disappear in your place, dear mom";
- Backache is a refusal to bow to the mother or father;
- Phantom pain is the need to take the removed organ into the heart (and perhaps the person it started to represent), and at the same time to accept the loss;
- Stomach problems are a dysfunctional attitude toward the mother;
- Psoriasis and atopic dermatitis are a curse—someone in the system is angry with their former partner;
- Headache and heartache are accumulated, suppressed love;
- Nausea is suppressed curses.

Despite these findings, the developer of systemic constellations remained open to new insights, as illustrated by his discussion with systemic therapist Gerhard Walper on autism:

Walper: In Garmisch you formulated the following hypothesis: the autist holds back a scream or a word. When this word or this scream is expressed, something opens in the soul. Love can flow again and the autist can perceive again and make contact.

Hellinger: Yes. I had had some experience with autists before and I wanted to test that in a constellation in Garmisch. The word the autistic child could not say in the constellation was "Mama." There are many different contexts here. In a course for psychotic people in Santa Barbara, there was also a family with autists. The constellation was very dramatic, and a new aspect surfaced here. One cannot reduce autism to a simple pattern, that would be far too primitive. The autist is someone who takes on himself something with love. [. . .] It often involves a criminal. But I do not reduce it to that. I remain alert and if something else comes up, I follow that. (Hellinger and Walper, n.d.)[6]

The patterns described by Hellinger really occur during constellations, but they must not be accepted as fixed and unambiguous, and even more so as comprehensive explanations. For the same disorder, there may be different constellations, and seemingly the same factors—for example, rejecting the mother—result in various dysfunctions. In addition, each constellation varies in details.

Exclusion and Entanglement

The most specific pathogenic process addressed by the theory of systemic constellations is entanglement, that is, unconscious identification with an older (earlier) member of the family. We are connected with a given person without knowing it—the entangled person looks internally at the older member of the family and follows him, imitating him in some aspect and desiring to share his fate. He can partially follow that person's life path or adopt his personality traits.

We use the term "entanglement" to refer to all cases of unconscious "joining" someone's fate. I would, however, distinguish two main types of entanglement: (1) related to a person one has never had contact with, and maybe even does not know about his existence, or (2) associated with a person important to us. In the first case, it is someone who had died or become absent in some other way before we were born: the elder brother or sister who died in childhood, the father's ex-partner. In the second case, it may be the parent, grandfather, older siblings, or siblings of parents, and sometimes the killer or victim. The root of the first type of entanglement is the exclusion of a given person from the family system. When someone is excluded, then someone else takes on himself that person's fate and becomes his representative in the system. In this way, he brings him back to the system as if he were saying, "You belong here too."

Entanglement exerts a very strong influence on the life of the entangled person. It alienates him from himself. Identification with another member of the system can be so strong that in a constellation he sees himself in another person's representative, not in the representative of himself. Wrong choices and failures in life, unsuccessful relationships, bad mood, and serious illnesses may be determined by entanglement. Identification with the excluded can take the form of creating one's own life so as to be excluded, wronged, beaten. The phrase "I am like you" reflects this identification.

The attempt to live a "double life" is at the same time carrying a double burden. It cannot be successful. Because entanglement concerns those whose fate was difficult, identification with them cannot have good consequences all the more.

The second type of entanglement may concern the people we have been in contact with, for example, our parents. There are two main dynamics here that can be expressed with the following words:

- "I'll follow you";
- "Rather me than you."

It is often a three-generational dynamics. "I'll follow you" is the script of the parent following, for example, his deceased sibling or parent, while "Rather me than you" is uttered by his child, wanting to stop him. These dynamics lead to diseases and suicides. They are based on the bond and need for balance and on magical thinking, according to which one can die for someone, keep him alive thanks to love, connect with someone through death, or shoulder someone's guilt. For example, someone who lost his father in childhood, says internally, "I'll follow you." He turns away from life, which takes the form of emotional absence, dullness of existence, diseases, or suicidal tendencies. In turn, his son unconsciously says, "Rather me than you" and blocks his own vitality, achievements, destroys his value by, for example, becoming a drug addict. In this way, he tries to pull his father away from the movement toward death or leaving the family. So he is governed by a kind of magical thinking that his defeat will somehow protect his father. Of course, neither the father nor the son is aware of their subconscious motives. Externally, both of them may make an impression that they are focused only on themselves and emotionally indifferent. The father may not be interested in the son too much, and the son may think ill of his father. Deep in the soul, however, they are directed by love.

Later in his work, Hellinger identified yet another sentence, expressed by an older member of the family, for example, by the mother, whose problems or depression her child wants to take on himself. This sentence reads: "Yes, you for me."

It means that the parent—unconsciously—agrees that the child will take over his difficulties. In constellations, we see it in situations where the parent wants to hide behind the child and pushes him, as it were, to the foreground, for example, in the face of something traumatic, which primarily concerns the parent, not the child. Standing behind the child, he does not have to look at it and follow it. This does not mean that the parent is self-serving and lacks love. It is possible to change this attitude in the course of a constellation—the parent's representative, sooner or later, becomes ready to confront the trauma. I understand this transformation as the potential readiness that was present in the parent from the beginning.

Violation of the Hierarchy

As I said above, the system has a hierarchy—the given direction of transmitting and taking of "psychological legacy." The existence of hierarchy is most clearly manifested when it is violated. Through the consequences borne by the one who puts himself not in his place.

The most frequent type of violation of the hierarchy is patronizing the parents. It may take an aggressive form when the child considers the parents to be "inferior," "less intelligent," or a caring one, which is called parentification and is a kind of role reversal in the parent-child relationship. At the systemic level, the disturbance of the parent-child hierarchy always works in the same way—it prevents development. Someone who violates the hierarchy and falsely puts himself above his parents, internally remains a "big child" and closes his path to development.

Violating the hierarchy usually provides a secondary gratification. The child that has violated the hierarchy feels exceptional, better, and with special rights. The fact that these feelings occur can be observed at workshops. The person starts to realize them the moment he is about to accept the hierarchy and suddenly feels that he may lose something. He confronts the fact that he will become someone ordinary, living an ordinary life. However, it is precisely the acceptance of this "ordinary life" that is a prerequisite for being able to achieve lasting and tangible successes in life. Otherwise, we will be left with illusory internal gratifications—an unjustified sense of being someone special.

Based on the example of parentification, one can explain what respect—a concept that is quite often referred to in systemic constellations—is. For parentification is associated with a lack of respect for the parent, although outwardly this may be difficult to notice. Take the following example: a woman looks after her father, cleans his apartment, brings him food, and medicines. This situation may seem to be purely positive—we could see here a concerned daughter taking care of her elderly parent. The woman advises her father, sometimes instructs him, treats him a bit patronizingly, but it is understandable in the face of his senile incapableness. However, if we take a closer look at her attitude, we can discover that she puts herself above her father. It could turn out that in her internal world this woman does not recognize the hierarchy, does not accept her father as a father, does not want to accept the fact that there is a level on which she is "small" and he is "big." She was the one who originally needed care, and he was her guardian. She was the one who entered his already formed life, not the other way round.

Violating the hierarchy is also influenced by the situational factors and the attitude of the parents. Sometimes the child replaces the parent's former partner or someone from his family of origin, or the parent addresses his needs to the child, although he should address them to his parents. Such an attitude, if it is manifested from the child's earliest years—when, for example, the abusive alcoholic or hysterical mother expects care from her several-year-old daughter—must lead to the reversal of the parent-child relationship. As a result of violation of the hierarchy, the development toward true adulthood withers. It cannot progress because in our own mind we have already reached the state of "adulthood."

Also in the hierarchy between siblings, the older siblings are more important than the younger—we receive from the older ones, we are more dependent on them. It seems to be particularly problematic if someone illegitimately occupies the first place among the siblings, that is, recognizes himself as the firstborn child, while there is an older half-sibling or when there had been a child who had died before he was born. Of course, the fact that he is unaware of the existence of those older siblings does not mean that the hierarchy remains intact.

Kleinian psychoanalyst Hanna Segal said that her older sister's death had a strong impact on her life:

> [. . .] although my sister was 4 when she died and therefore older than I was, to me she was always a younger sister. I was very taken up in analysis with being very inhibited in my ambition whenever I found myself in a situation of competition with sister figures. I can remember running in races, getting towards the head of the file and then just falling back as soon as I got nearer the finishing line. (Quinodoz 2008, 4)

Segal interprets the above relationship as "survivor guilt." Of course, in constellations, we also observe such processes, but in this case, it could have been an unconscious need to respect the hierarchy. While running, Segal usurped the precedence and at the same time gave it up regularly. In this way, she unconsciously returned to the proper hierarchy ("You are the first"). My clients faced very similar situations. If someone illegitimately took the first place, he was constantly "the second," wasted opportunities, was never on time, or was preempted. Despite the belief that "it belongs to me," that "this place is mine."

The Interrupted Movement of Love

The interrupted movement of love (German *unterbrochene Hinbewegung*), or the interrupted movement toward the mother or father is a kind of internal separation of the child from the parent. The child's natural state is to be open to his parents, but because of their emotional or physical absence, he can inwardly block them out. The reason may be the hospitalization of the parent or child in the early years of his life, the parent's death or depression. This kind of separation causes a psychological pain that can turn into a hostile attitude toward the parents. Back, heart and headaches, anxiety, and depression may occur. The interrupted movement toward the mother, which consists in turning away from her internally, results in difficulties both in relationships and at work. It is due to the fact that this condition impairs the ability to take, which translates into an inability to use what life offers us. The mother is the first person who gives us, the first we want to take from. If this desire is blocked because of a grudge, the ability to take good things will also be blocked. That is why our relationships will become asymmetrical, we will try to prove to ourselves and others that we do not need anything or we will only be able to give, which will result in growing frustration.

Interruption of the child's primal movement toward the mother may take place as early as in the perinatal period. Melanie could not enter a lasting relationship, she broke up her relationships and suffered because of that. The most important thing in her constellation was that she could not accept her mother, and even wanted to reject her. The words: "It's hard for me to accept you" were too weak. "I don't want anything to do with you" did not express her attitude either. That is why I suggested the following words: "I'd like to get you out of my heart." The client fully agreed with that. After she said those words, I—as a representative of her mother—moved away spontaneously, and the client felt "like a four-year-old child who forgot the kindergarten bag." She was defenseless and lost. Before, she had seemed to continue to hold onto her attitude. What appeared now enabled us to proceed. I assumed the early period, probably the birth, was crucial here. I asked Melanie to lie down on a blanket and told her she was an infant now. Representing the mother, I did not feel any attraction toward the child, I could not embrace her and give her warmth.

This made me think about the mother's mother. I put an object representing the mother next to the client, and I stood as the grandmother. I immediately held my stomach and bent forwards, as if I had a strong pain in this area. I asked Melanie if she knew anything about her mother's birth. I suspected that she did not know anything about it, but she said that her mother had been born in the seventh month of pregnancy, it had been a very difficult birth, and she had remained in an incubator for a long time. During delivery, the memory of each mother's own birth and early relationship with her mother is activated. Due to the trauma of birth, which primarily involved separation from the mother, the client's mother was unable to accept her own child. In addition, Melanie was born by caesarean section. This early interruption of the movement of love caused that Melanie emotionally blocked her mother out and rejected her. She highlighted many of her mother's harming behaviors, but she was unaware that the basic trauma was rooted in the time of birth. All the more she did not think it could be her mother's birth. Now, lying on her side, with her mother's representative and the symbolic representation of her grandmother behind, she could finally understand her history and open herself to her mother. It brought her peace. She said, "I'm complete now."

Refusal to Accept Parents

Refusal to internally honor parents (accept "parents as parents") is the cause of many life and health problems. Hellinger maintains that it may even be the cause of cancer. Not accepting one or both parents worsens one's mood (while acknowledging them immediately increases the level of energy and improves well-being). These phenomena are independent of our will, working automatically. As in many other psychic dynamics discovered by Hellinger, there is a kind of dialectic and interpenetration of apparent contradictions here as well. The rejection of a parent often results in an intense unconscious attempt to imitate him. A typical example is a son of an alcoholic who, together with his mother, negates his father's value, and then becomes an alcoholic himself (the rejection of the parent by the child is dictated by loyalty to the other parent who does not honor the first one).

We are often not aware that we reject our parents. It seems to us that we have a "good relationship" with them and that "everything is fine." A constellation can show us, however, that things look different. Even a simple sentence can reveal our difficulty in accepting parents: the client cannot say to the representative of the father (mother): "You are my father" ("You are my mother"). The difference between declarations and what can be seen in the constellation results from the fact that during the constellation we can face the "essence" of the parent and be confronted with the core of our relationship with him.

Atonement—Pseudo-Balance

In our psyche, there is a balancing mechanism. When we receive something, we want to give something. And when we hurt someone, we want to be punished. If punishment does not come, we impose penance on ourselves. The person who does penance inflicts punishment on himself in the hope that it will balance his guilt. Atonement can be suffering, illness, failures, accidents, or suicide. All these events, though usually considered to be accidental, may in fact be expected, because they give hope for a balance. However, it will not be the balance concordant with the orders of love. This pseudo-balance is destructive in the long run, in addition, it makes two persons suffer instead of one.

There is something more about atonement. It often results from the unwillingness to accept the blame. Whoever cannot face his guilt, who desires to keep a clear conscience forever, atones. Atonement is sometimes associated with refusal to establish a relationship with the victim and reluctance to face him in one's inner world. It is easier to blame oneself, to be unhappy, and thus to achieve an apparent balance, than to confront the truth about oneself and give the victim his rightful place. The true balance can be a sincere thank-you, or simply accepting some person and event, looking at them and expressing regret with the words, "I am sorry." It may seem strange, but some prefer to die than to do it. This happens in the course of some diseases, for example, cancer in some women—they prefer to die with a "clear conscience" than to accept their blame, which may be, for instance, an abortion.

Generally speaking, atonement is caused by situations such as not accepting a parent, doing great harm to someone, aborting a child, but also the feeling that one gained unjustly, because, for instance, he was his parents' favorite child. Both something that was the real cause of our deeds and something that we had no influence on, such as a miscarriage or giving birth to a disabled child, can be felt as guilt. Even a fortunate event, for example, surviving a catastrophe, can be experienced as guilt and demand a balance.

Double Shift

Alexandra's problem was her great anger toward her husband. Their relationship had been bad for a long time, her husband wanted to divorce her, then he changed his mind and they were supposed to rebuild the relationship, but they could not manage. Recently, Alexandra felt cheated, even used, which made her furious. I had no idea what I could do to heal that relationship, especially that I was working with just one of the spouses. I focused on identifying what should be positioned in the constellation. I asked Alexandra herself to stand in the constellation, and another person to represent "what aroused her anger/was related to that anger." The client felt that she wanted to beat, hit, and kick. The representative of the "anger" stood calmly and watched. At one point, she said, "I feel strong." Those words made the client even more angry, and I associated them with what she told me about her husband. The "anger" was a representation of him. The client was still beating and kicking, but—from the very beginning—she was not doing it in the direction of the representative, but chaotically and in all directions. I put a pillow as "this what she was really hitting." The client hit the pillow gently and then began to look at it.

I stood on the pillow as a representative of that "something." I immediately smiled at Alexandra spontaneously and she smiled back. She said she saw me as a baby, and I sat down after a while. I asked who it could be. "My brother," she replied. The child who was not born, he was aborted. The client's anger was her mother's suppressed anger toward her father for demanding the abortion. It was the so-called "double shift," that is, shifting the anger to another subject and object—the anger passed on from the mother to the daughter and was directed toward her husband, not her father. Although I had talked to her for a long time, it had not crossed my or her mind that the cause of her problem could have had its roots in that matter.

ELEMENTS OF THE THERAPY PROCESS

Therapeutic Objectives and Interventions

The strategic goal of Hellinger's therapy is to reveal "what is" in the family system and to bring about the orders of love. The latter involves a few key interventions:

- Including the excluded, whose identification and repositioning in the system is the primary objective of the therapy. Hellinger argues that family constellations are first of all aimed at connecting what has been separated. It turns out that including those who influence the members of the system through the bond and are not remembered or the system members are unaware of their existence, brings a huge reduction in tension as well as peace and strength. This is revealed in a constellation even when such people are victims or killers, that is, the persons who are normally perceived as causing pain or horror.
- Bringing the bonds to light, that is, uncovering childlike love for the family system members, even those who are consciously condemned or considered to be unimportant. Revealing archaic fantasies, related to this bond, about saving someone from death through one's own sacrifice, about atoning for him, and so on.
- Changing identification into a relation—by standing face to face (with the help of representatives) with those with whom there is an unconscious bond and unconscious identification. Also leaving what "is theirs" and not ours with them, such as a hard lot or a desire to take revenge. As a result of these actions, the entanglement gets resolved. Being "with someone" replaces being "like him."
- Facilitating the client's reconciliation with his parents. Our psyche perceives them as a necessary beginning of our life. The parents are also the "gateway" to taking strength from the ancestors, the flow of which is blocked if we internally reject them.
- Restoring the hierarchy that everyone in the system unconsciously desires to submit to, although it is sometimes unconsciously violated. A constellation makes it possible to rebuild it, thus to find one's right place in the system.
- Leading the client to the point where he lets the members of the family system go if they are unstoppably drawn to death or to leave the family. This

means that he abandons the self-destructive and futile attempts to restrain someone in their movement, respecting their individual fate.

- Enabling the client to restore the interrupted movement of love toward his mother or father. In a constellation, this movement can be restored with the help of the representative of the parent, through the act of slowly approaching him and internally opening up to one's childlike need for a bond with the parent. The child existing in the client renews his relationship with him because he never stopped needing it.

Other therapeutic interventions include strengthening gender identification by placing the man by his father (in the male line) and the woman—by her mother (in the female line); unburdening the child by moving him away from his systemically burdened parent and positioning him by the other parent; placing the stillborn children by their siblings; placing the aborted children (usually in a sitting position) by their parents; restoring the hierarchy (for example, ending parentification by saying: "I am only a child"); enabling one to resign from atonement through the acceptance of blame and "looking into the eyes of the one who paid the price"; enabling one to thank and develop a sense of gratitude instead of demands and assessments (by bowing down, accepting, saying "Thank you"); showing that someone was identified with another person (e.g., the child represented his parent's former partner); confronting the victims and perpetrators (e.g., by placing the perpetrator next to the victim); showing the hidden relationship with the perpetrator of sexual abuse; enabling support from the previous generations (by positioning the ancestors behind the client).

Sentences of Strength

Sentences of strength (German *Sätze der Kraft*) are—next to repositioning of the representatives in space—a basic element of therapeutic intervention. They lead to changes in the system and the client's attitude. Sentences of strength are suggested by the therapist and spoken by the representatives or the clients. Sometimes the representatives themselves come up with them, because—captivated by the movement of the constellation—they feel what is right and become the ones who express the orders of love. Sentences of strength are to show the bond, restore the hierarchy, and give back one's responsibility. Basically, they are a relatively closed catalog and one does not have to create them anew. However, certain modifications or changes in emphases are often appropriate (sometimes sentences are modified by the representatives or the clients themselves, if they feel that a slightly different form is more adequate).

It is surprising how universal sentences of strength are. Common experience with language teaches us that there are as many meanings as there are people—everyone understands it in their own way. However, sentences of strength invariably produce the same effect, no one questions them, everyone understands their meaning. Of course, this is not only because of their simplicity and content relating to the most important human affairs but also because of the context in which they are uttered. In a context such as the confrontation with one's own family system, they have a lasting transformative effect. Therefore, the seemingly pathetic term "sentences of strength" is fully justified and deeply accurate.

There are two basic types of sentences that are uttered by the representatives or the client during the constellation: resolving the problem and showing it. The first are sentences of strength in the strict sense. The latter are sentences of strength only partially, but they also have a therapeutic effect. For example, the client says to his mother's representative, "Dear mom, thank you for my life. I leave what's yours with you, with respect." This is a sentence that solves the problem, because in this way the client leaves the infantile attempts to save the mother and suffer instead of her. We suggest the sentences that show the problem when the client cannot say a sentence of resolution, because he is evidently blocked. For example, it may be difficult for him to leave the problem with his father or mother because of his persistent belief in magical solutions or because of fear of loneliness. It may also be difficult for him to accept his parent because of a persistent grudge. In this case, we ask the client to say, "I can't take you as a father for now." This sentence does not stiffen the client's attitude, but it is still a step toward accepting the father. Sometimes saying such words causes that the internal process starts, which in time leads the given person to accept the parent. It also happens that during the constellation, the client's attitude changes and a sentence of resolution becomes possible.

Sometimes a sentence of resolution can be a sentence that seemingly ties the client to the problem even more. In a constellation of one of the clients, Sarah, we touched many spheres related to the family secrets. The initial interview also showed that many things in her family were hidden and ignored in order to preserve the apparent conformity with the requirements of religion. In the course of the constellation—in which we used a number of figurines representing the members of her family—the client slowly gained a sense of peace and unburdening. However, when her figurine stood opposite the whole family, and I asked her to say, "I leave what's yours with you, with respect," she did not feel good. She said it seemed to her that everything was "left unfinished."

It surprised me that someone reacted this way to—after all—bringing about order. I knew that it was definitely not "chaos," as the client called it. I suggested that she say: "I'll take something from each of you, a part of your fate. And I'll carry it further into the future. With love." After saying this sentence, the client felt good and complete. If it had been a sentence just showing the problem, it would have worked as a paradoxical intervention, that is, it would have indicated an incorrect attitude. In this case, it was a resolving sentence. Liberation from carrying something "that is not mine" became possible through the acceptance and gesture of conscious consent to what comes from the family. In this way, Sarah could fully honor the bond with the family members.

If one can valuate it at all, then the sentence of strength that expresses the most of the essence of constellations is "You have a place in my heart. I leave your fate with you, with respect." It shows how systemic constellations connect what may seem separate: the bond and autonomy. This sentence contains an affirmation of the bond as well as the process of emancipation. It respects the deep love we have for the family system members, and at the same time frees us and enables us to go into our individual lives. I take someone into my heart, that is, I confirm my bond, and at the same time I leave his fate with him, which means I gain freedom.

This double move is a way out of the entanglement. If we wanted to resolve the entanglement by saying: "I leave your fate with you, I don't want to have anything to do with you," there would be a movement toward identification with the given person. Similarly, if we only confirmed the bond: "I'm tied to you and your fate," we could even strengthen the client's incorrect identification (although in some situations, this sentence could show the problem and initiate the process of change). Adding the phrase "with respect" means that we actually consider the other person, we are not driven by anger against him.

Here are other examples of sentences of resolution: "You are the first, I am the second" (second wife to first wife); "I loved your father very much, and if you become like him, I assent to that" (divorced woman to her children, who hate their father); "I am sorry. Now I give you a place in my heart" (parent to aborted child); "She is my mother and I am her daughter. I have nothing to do with your ex-wife" (daughter to father, who identifies the daughter with his ex-wife); "Look, I have become just like you, and I am content with that" (daughter to her mother when she is afraid she will become like her); "Dear mother, even though you have lost your life because of my birth, it must not be in vain. In remembrance of you, I will make something of my life" (child to his mother who died in childbirth); "Dear father, even if you go, I will stay, and I honor you as my father" (child to his father who wants to leave, die); "I will bear it myself. As far as I am concerned, you are free" (suffering father to his daughter who wants to follow him); "What you did was bad for me and I am leaving you with the consequences. I will make something of my life in spite of what happened" (child to his parents who did him wrong); "We gladly gave you life and gladly did for you everything that we did. We let you go now, in peace. Yet for us you will always remain our child and we your parents" (parents to their child who died); "Dear father, within me you are still alive. I will let you participate in what I do" (daughter to her father who committed suicide).

These sentences do not have to be identical to the ones I have mentioned, but they always underline the bond, autonomy, memory, and contain acknowledgment of one's own place and responsibility, along with giving back the place and responsibility of others.

Representatives

The function of representatives is the most important one in constellations. Paradoxically, it is also the simplest. There is no specific instruction for a representative other than "Follow your movement." Sometimes one does not even have to say that much, even if a given person participates in a constellation for the first time (it is enough to bring the person "into the field"). It is this complete lack of orienting the representatives that underlies the enormous strength of constellations. Spontaneous movement and sensations in the body are the most important phenomena that occur in constellations. They appear completely regardless of the will and thinking of the representatives. Feelings are a bit lower on the scale of importance, and thoughts—which the representatives turn into words—are scaled even lower. Experience shows that all phenomena that spontaneously occur in constellations (feelings, thoughts, visualizations, and so on) are significant, but the movement and sensations in the body are the most solid basis for the constellation. They are the energy that directs the constellation and protects from the misleading influence of reasoning, concluding, and fantasizing.

Representatives often experience symptoms that correspond to the diseases of the people they represent. These sensations often appear suddenly, immediately after entering the role and are not invoked in any conscious way. Take the example of a constellation of a young man, Matthew, who suffered an unaccountable paralysis of one side of the body. The paralysis receded, but the man had to continue the treatment. His mother present in the constellation session made a mistake and said it was the right side of the body. However, Matthew's representative (a woman) clearly felt that something was happening to her left side, which was consistent with the fact.

Movement in constellations is initiated by the knowing field, which takes place completely beyond the sphere of thinking of the representatives. One can also see it clearly when we bring a person important to the system in a constellation. The representatives immediately experience an impulse, a feeling, and their mood changes straightaway. These phenomena occur before any reflection. In a constellation, the representatives reflect the knowledge, which is not accessible for the represented person. However, this is not random or irrelevant information, but information about things that are significant from a systemic point of view. The representatives, governed by the family field, which aims at order in the system, also express the orders of love—they unwittingly suggest words and gestures that introduce this order. Even those who do not know systemic constellations and have never participated in them before do it. This is one of the most amazing phenomena, confirming the universality and adequacy of the processes discovered by Hellinger.

VARIANTS OF THE TECHNIQUE AND METHOD

New Family Constellations

The first systemic constellations facilitated by Hellinger were quite directive. He moved the representatives a bit like pawns on a chessboard, asking them how they felt in a given configuration. Thanks to this information and his intuition and insights, he discovered respective systemic orders. With time, however, as a therapist, he gradually withdrew from the setting up process, giving room for spontaneous movements of the representatives.

Hellinger referred to the modification of the original technique of constellations as "movements of the soul" (by the term "soul" he meant the force that rules and guides living beings). The movements of the soul are a technique in which the representatives remain silent, and the therapist hardly intervenes, relying on the teleological aspect of constellations, that is, the self-existent movement of the system toward order.

Later, referring to mass and social processes, Hellinger began to speak of the "Great Soul," going beyond the boundaries of the family and connecting with other groups, and ultimately with all nature. Finally, he popularized the concept of "movements of the Spirit"[7] (German *Bewegungen des Geistes*). These changes are related to Hellinger's distinguishing of the spiritual conscience, that is, the strength or dynamics that aims at reconciliation. Hellinger says:

> The one who comes into harmony with the movements of the Spirit, can do nothing but turn to everyone equally, with benevolence and love, whatever their fate is. This love knows no boundaries. The spiritual conscience overcomes the distinctions between better and worse, between good and bad. (Hellinger 2008, 64)[8]

Having focused his interest on the movement of the Spirit, Hellinger introduced the term "Spiritual Family Constellations." He based them on the observation that a constellation develops as if it were guided by a force that connects everyone, leading to the disappearance of the distinction between better and worse, victims and perpetrators. Currently, family spiritual constellations are referred to as New Family Constellations (there are also other terms: "Medial Family Constellations," "Silent Family Constellations").

Silent family constellations, however, are based on the same laws and processes as constellations in which we use utterances of representatives. Sometimes they can deepen the ongoing process because movement can take us further than words that sometimes inhibit movement. But in other cases, words, especially in the form of sentences of strength, prove to be helpful to clients. They are also indispensable when working individually, without a group (see below).

Hellinger said, however, that old family constellations are over. How should we understand it? As a development of Hellinger himself, rather than deflating the therapeutic significance of the previously used technique. Besides, the work of today's therapists who use the so-called "classic technique" is not identical to Hellinger's early work. With his growing experience and development of intuition, Hellinger was often able to get to the heart of the problem, even before starting the constellation. He also concentrated on shorter interventions, with fewer representatives, that is, he brought only the most important people in the constellation. Sometimes he did not start the constellation at all, but gave the client a word or a sentence that, containing the essence of the problem, had a transformative effect. He described this process in the following way:

> I focus inside. I open up to this person as he is, without knowing anything about him and without asking him, and I wait until I get a hint from somewhere else. It is often just a word or a short sentence. I ask this person to close his eyes. Then I say this word and this sentence and ask him to let it have an effect on him. This word or this sentence cannot be derived from any idea. It is suggested and presented to me from somewhere else. (Hellinger 2014a, 179–80)[9]

New family constellations have their own aesthetics and style, but this does not mean that they are more helpful to clients. There are clients for whom the classic technique will be better, and on the other hand, there are cases when it is good to ask representatives to be silent and follow only their movement. The latter can take place, for example, when we see that great traumas from the past play a part, such as war murders. Then it may be important to let them be expressed in silence, let the representatives be caught by a wide movement connecting the victims and perpetrators. Even in these cases, however, words do not have to be an obstacle, but an important complement. For instance, during a workshop in 2008, Hellinger gave the representatives the opportunity to talk about their feelings after the constellation and said that he saw "how important it is to give those participating in the constellation the opportunity to say what they have experienced" (Hellinger 2014, 48).[10]

There is no conflict between "new" and "classic" systemic constellations. In this book, writing mainly about classic family constellations, I do not have in mind the original form of Hellinger's work, but a technique that is based on both the earlier and later forms of his work.

Individual Constellations

Individual systemic constellations do not involve a group of representatives, it is the client-therapist work. They include

- Inner constellations, or visualizations;
- Constellations with special miniature figures or other objects (markers) representing elements of the system, which are placed on the table;
- Constellations with sheets of paper or objects denoting elements of the system, which are laid on the floor.

These constellations are more comprehensively described in chapter 2.

Structural Constellations

Structural constellations do not concentrate on family dynamics but on analyzing and solving diverse problems (Sparrer 2006; Varga and Sparrer 2018). The conflicting parties, client's questions, and possible solutions can be represented in them. The authors of this method, Matthias Varga von Kibéd and Insa Sparrer, understand the structural constellation as a form of language (transverbal language) in which one can find out deeper connections and background of a given problem through the verbal expressions and bodily sensations of a group of representatives.

In this technique, the tetralemma is used—a scheme derived from the logico-epistemological tradition of India. The tetralemma consists of four positions that can be described as: "the one," "the other," "both," and "neither of the two" (affirmation, negation, both, neither). Representatives take each of the four positions that are potential answers to a problem or question. Their feelings and feelings of the one who asks are the components of the answer. In addition, the fifth position (nonposition) is used, which can be called "something completely different." It leads the one who asks to a higher level, by suggesting a complete change of the client's attitude toward the problem.

Conceptual and Archetypal Constellations

Conceptual constellations have been developed by Joy Manné (Manné 2013). These are nonpersonal constellations concerning certain model situations. They enable one to observe general regularities occurring in systems. In this way one can, for example, check Hellinger's concise expression: "Men are bigger." What is behind it? Is it just a reference to the obvious? Or to some gender inequality? Manné writes:

> I divided the group into men and women and had them face each other in two lines. When a woman felt ready, she could approach a man and tell him, "You are bigger and I am smaller, and I agree." Every step of her approach had to be mindful, and her utterance had to convince the man. If it didn't, he told her and she repeated the exercise.
>
> When the exercise was well done, the man radiated joy, delight, warmth, relief, protection, love, desire, confidence, and more toward the woman. Those simple words evoked feelings the women had longed to experience coming from a man. The man too was happy. The acknowledgement made the man feel safe with the woman. It opened his heart and enabled him to stand in his manly strength and power in front of the woman, at last.
>
> As the men's and women's reactions showed, the exercise didn't take anything away from the woman. Rather, the man saw her as a valuable equal and partner. It did not disempower the woman while empowering the man. It empowered both equally. (Manné 2013, chap. 8)

Some therapists practice archetypal constellations in which archetypal figures and abstract concepts, such as a "shadow," "wisdom," "love," "freedom," and other, appear as elements of the system. However, one should remember that if there are many abstractions and general concepts, we depart from the essence of family constellations, in which relationships with concrete persons are most important.

Inspiration: The Constellation of the Intention

Franz Ruppert developed a method which he refers to as the constellation of the intention. In this method, the client expresses an intention, which he formulates in the form of a specific sentence. It can be a desire to discover the causes of some symptom or problem. A representative, selected from among the workshop participants, is assigned to each word from the client's sentence. Each "word" and the dynamics of the whole sentence that emerged between the representatives carry information about what happens in the client's psyche. Rupert also uses "trauma constellations," arguing that what underlies most symptoms and problems is a trauma, early trauma in particular, which results in states of mental dissociation. During the constellation, through representing, the original traumatic situation is recalled and enacted again, this time in a very conscious way. This helps to reintegrate the client's psyche (Ruppert 2012; Ruppert et al. 2016).

It must be pointed out, however, that Ruppert's method greatly deviates from Hellinger's systemic constellations. Its author does not recognize the orders of love, which precludes it from being regarded as systemic constellations. On the other hand, the method is so similar to constellations, from which it derives, that it needs to be mentioned.

NOTES

1. Some people claim that systemic constellations are not a psychotherapeutic method, which cannot be considered true. Constellations contain all the necessary elements of psychotherapy, such as the theory of development of disorders, clearly defined goals of therapeutic interventions, the clearly defined position and role of the therapist; they require a personal commitment from the client and involve his mental and emotional work. Last but not least, this method makes it possible to successfully eliminate mental suffering, behavioral, and psychosomatic disorders. At the end of his work, Bert Hellinger said that systemic constellations go beyond psychotherapy and suggested, that they should not be equated with it. He argued that constellations developed within psychotherapy, but this became an obstacle to their development, as many of the principles of psychotherapy do not apply to this method and what is more, they are against life itself. For these reasons, he referred to them as "Life help" (German *Lebenshilfe*). Ultimately, whether or not we consider constellations to be psychotherapy depends solely on how we define it.
2. I use the term "client" because in the case of constellations, it is more adequate than the term "patient," which suggests a very asymmetrical relationship with the therapist.
3. Quotation translated from Polish.
4. All the clients' names and identifying details have been changed in the book.
5. This is the opinion of Bert Hellinger himself, although in his late work he seemed to treat early deaths, abortions, and miscarriages equally.
6. Quotation translated from German.
7. Also referred to as the movements of the Spirit-Mind.
8. Quotation translated from German.
9. Quotation translated from German.
10. Quotation translated from Polish.

Chapter 2

Elements of Therapeutic Practice

INDIVIDUAL CONSTELLATIONS

The original constellation technique is working with the help of a group. We have at our disposal a few, a dozen, or even dozens of people who can become representatives of one's family members. We use their sensitivity, faculty of insight, and visualization. When I work with representatives, in most cases, I follow their suggestions, and this always proves fruitful.

Individual systemic constellations are grounded on the same general principles as group ones. Only the work technique is different. The basic techniques in individual constellations are the use of figurines and sheets of paper laid on the floor. In the first case, we work on the table, in the second—in space and with the whole body. Two other techniques are working with imagination (visualization), or internal constellations, and what I define as self-constellations.

There are many ways to work with one's imagination. One of them—active imagination—was proposed by Carl Gustav Jung (Samuels et al. 2013). At first, a person concentrates on a mood, image, dream, event, or place in space. Then comes a chain of images and associations that begin to live their own lives and develop according to their own logic. According to Jung, this type of daydreaming made contact with the archetypal unconscious possible. Internal constellations, just as this technique, use the fact that the images have their own movement.

During the exercise, the client can imagine, for example, where his parents would stand in relation to him. One of my clients visualized that her mother was very close to her and she felt very uncomfortable about it. That short exercise revealed her feeling of being trapped and difficulty in accepting her as a mother, which was fully confirmed in the course of her long-term psychotherapy.

Similarly, if the client imagines the father standing in front of him and tries to look him in the eye, then the father's face, his look, his posture, or distance from the client will not be an expression of his projection but will bring objectified knowledge about the father and the relationship with him. The son may notice that his father is not looking at him. This looking at something else will not be a fantasy of the son who felt underestimated by his father, but an indication that the father is actually looking in a different direction, being probably unconsciously bound to some person. Also, one's difficulty in imagining a given person will point to his incomplete presence due to entanglement rather than the inability of the client himself to imagine pictures or persons (Franke 2003, 116–17).

We can also meet internally with our grandparents and great-grandparents. We do not need to know their faces or know anything about them. It is enough to recall them in our minds, for instance, as "the grandfather's father on the distaff side." We can then observe our psychophysical reactions, such as changes in our mood or pulse rate, which can be surprising.

The therapist can also use his own imagination to understand the client. When, for example, I imagine his mother and father behind the client, or actually when I simply try to "see" them behind him, I will "see" the persons in a specific configuration—closer or farther from the client, big or small, standing, lying, or maybe cringing. These imageries will not be my projections but will express some rudimentary aspects of the client's relationship with his parents.

Constellations with figurines were initiated by therapist Jacob Schneider, who used his son's Playmobil figurines and began to arrange client families from them. Some, instead of figurines, use wooden blocks that have no arms or legs, they only have a "face" (marked viewing direction), gender (square or round in shape), and age (small and large blocks). Anyway, any items can be used that have one side different, that is, the viewing direction is marked. The simplest type of marker will be a cup with its lid turned upside down.

The client sets up the picture of his family. Next, he is asked about the feelings that each of the figurines might have in its place and whether he sees in them a "desire" to move. If so, he moves the figurine accordingly. Questions about feelings or movements of the inanimate figurines are only seemingly absurd, clients easily accept this convention of work, and their feelings about individual figurines are usually clear. Looking at the figurines, they identify that someone is sad, someone else feels lonely, someone else—angry. They have the feeling that someone represented by a figurine does not feel comfortable in their place, wants to change it, get close to someone, or move away from someone. The therapist also perceives the knowing field connected with the figurines. The way the therapist perceives "emotions" and "movements" of the figurines generally coincides with how the client perceives them.

These plastic figurines, when we ascribe them given identities, bring us information that cannot be obtained in a typical conversation. This information sometimes concerns the matters of which the client had no knowledge. For example, that he has unknown siblings or that his grandfather is bound to a deceased person. Also in this kind of work, the most important is the influence of the knowing field, which is manifested, inter alia, in the fact that the client ascribes to individual figurines the emotions and attitudes that are different from those he knew before.

Apart from working with figurines, another very effective technique is the technique of using sheets of paper or other objects put on the floor, which are to represent people from the system (or impersonal elements such as "work" and "problem"). Although he preferred group work, Hellinger also worked this way. He set up shoes that symbolized given persons and stood next to them with the client, thanks to this both of them could feel what the represented person felt. We now know that one does not need to use such specific items, as sheets of paper marked as "father," "mother," "father's father," and so on are enough. The therapist begins to represent each person, standing on each sheet of paper one by one. The constellation goes in a sequential manner. First, "I am," for example, the "mother." In this role I feel, I move spontaneously, sometimes I communicate my condition to the client. Then I leave the role of the "mother" and move to the next role. Then the next. Finally, I stand as the "mother" again. Sometimes I repeat the cycle several times, making the constellation progress this way. Usually, during this work, I add more sheets, for instance, representing the "cause of what is happening to the mother" or "this what the father is looking at."

It is worth mentioning that when I represent the client's loved ones, such as his father, mother, husband, or wife, in the vast majority of cases, the client immediately recognizes well-known behaviors or characteristic movements.

I use the double perspective all the time—of the representative and the therapist. Experiencing someone's uncertainty, fear or tears springing to my eyes, at the same time, I ask the client calmly what he feels, what is happening to him at a given moment. I let the feelings of people from his system govern me, but I remember to continue my task as a therapist. During this work, I can also use visualizations—for example, as the client's father, I stand in my imagination in front of his parents (the client's grandparents). Obviously, they are not any visions, but a kind of "semi-images," a feeling that the given person exists and some elementary information about his attitude, seeing him as strong or weak, giving love, feeling lost, bound to someone else. The client, although he remains only an observer, experiences strong feelings when he stands in the field of systemic forces, and this affects his psychophysical state. At the end of the session, I propose sentences of strength, bowing or standing in the string of generations. Then the feeling of unburdening, leaving the weight, and a characteristic spontaneous breath of relief appear.

I have been asked many times what is better—a group or individual constellation. There is no answer. Perhaps a group constellation is better if someone was adopted and had no contact with his parents. In this case, contact with the representatives of his biological parents, a woman and a man, will be more touching for him. In turn, an individual constellation from the very beginning demands that the client be fully involved.

I refer to constellations unassisted by others as self-constellations. An example is the constellation during which I worked on my allergy. I placed the first object (a bottle for watering flowers) on the floor as my "allergy." This constellation made me realize that the disease was actually a manifestation of my bond with someone from my ancestral system, and that its symptoms, such as lacrimation, were unconscious crying. After this exercise I became free from the allergy.

In this way, one can test various relationships and a deeper level of one's attitude toward the partner. We can only use our imagination, assuming that the given person is standing in front of us. Then we can check what movement appears in us, how we see the other person, what move he seems to be making. The next step in this work is to represent another person to oneself. We give ourselves a self-suggestion that we "leave" ourselves in a given place, we put there an object that will represent us, and we stand as the other person. Interestingly, even if we have certain wishes and ideas about the other person and the relationship with him, reaching objective cognition is not difficult. Even if the obtained knowledge contradicts our expectations, the objective movement will be clear and stronger than our wishes. Of course, this exercise should only be performed by people who are sufficiently trained in constellations and ready to exceed their wishful thinking.

UNEXPECTED OUTCOMES OF THE SIMPLE PROCEDURE

Systemic constellations amaze. Despite the unusually simple procedure, during their course, there are phenomena whose existence cannot be deduced from ordinary psychological knowledge or life experience. The most unusual is probably the very possibility of accessing the information about the client and his family system. It is enough that the therapist faces the client as, for example, his father's representative, and the knowledge about the client's relationship with his father is quickly deepened—not only the therapist's knowledge, but also the client's. It is enough to place an object next to the client that represents his brother, thus pointing to the system hierarchy, to reveal the client's hidden attitude or feelings that he was not aware of (grievance, jealousy, love, and so on).

Spectacular is the strength with which clients experience this simple procedure, which is particularly evident during an individual session, where the therapist is the only representative. In this case, one could imagine that the person who comes to a session for the first time and does not know what to expect will regard the therapist's movement, grimaces, or lying on the floor as a bizarre, perhaps even embarrassing, show. Nothing like that. Activating the field of the client's family always leads to clear psychophysical feelings, and the person who takes part in the constellation clearly sees that these are matters that concern him.

I also do not think that anyone could assume that they will react with their whole body to setting up a few plastic figurines and that the session will have a decisive impact on curing their long-lasting illness. However, this is what actually happens. Representing the important family members, even in the form of small figures, triggers processes that are incomparable to the tool used. The client experiences tingling sensations, chest tightness, leg tremor, and many other physical symptoms as well as strong emotions. At the end, he is overcome with a psychophysical sense of relief. This state can be compared to the situation where someone learns that a very stressful situation has been solved successfully. The relief is usually accompanied by an involuntary deep breath, often occurring before it becomes consciously noticed, which is another proof that we deal with unconscious factors here.

Without the experience provided by a constellation, the effect of sentences of strength and simple gestures, such as bowing, is impossible to predict. Saying in the right moment to the representative of the father, who transferred the emotions from his mother to his daughter: "I'm just a child," has an immediate unburdening effect, and the effect is permanent. The same applies, for instance, to bowing before the fate of the ancestors, accompanied by the intention to "leave what belongs to the past in the past"—there is a change that is felt psychophysically, and in the relationships with the family and in life something starts to work better.

When the therapist or a member of the workshop group represents the client, it often happens that he experiences painful emotions that the client was unaware of, as they had been deeply repressed. In such cases, they are released as if *per procura* by the representative, which the client feels very clearly. The client does not experience this in the form of similarly negative feelings, but in the vast majority of cases in the form of a feeling of calm that fills him. The fact that someone took on himself his pain and showed it brings an immediate drop in tension and a feeling of relief. As if the negative feelings were something material, and the representative became a vent through which they could escape. If we told the average person raised in Western culture that such processes are not only possible, but during the session are the norm, they would certainly not believe it.

Jacob's older sister died when she was two months old. He told me about it only when her existence became apparent in the constellation. The session revealed that Jacob was perceived by his mother as if he had been a girl. Why did the mother not notice the boy in him? In my opinion, because it would have amounted to admitting that her first child was dead. And indeed, representing her, I was not able to say, "My daughter died." At first Jacob was angry with his mother for not seeing him. However, when he uttered the sentences of strength, that he was a boy and left with his mother what was hers—that is, her difficulty in experiencing mourning—he felt a blockade. In fact, he wanted to help his mother and be that child for her.

When he stood in line with the objects representing his siblings, I asked him to say, "I'm second, I'm a son, I'm a boy." He misspoke twice. He said that "I'm a sister" came to his mind. Earlier he had not had the slightest idea of these connections, he had not realized that his mother had seen him as a girl, and he had not thought of himself as a "substitute" sister. A few minutes of work and a person "playing" his mother was enough to make these deep attitudes see the light of day.

If something is inconsistent with the orders of love in the constellation, the representatives immediately sense it. This sensitivity is completely unusual and results from the effect of the family field.

During a constellation, Melissa confronted with the fact that she badly needed her deceased father and his support. She said to his representative, "You always interceded for me." However, at that moment, the father's representative stepped back. There was something in her attitude and words that violated the orders of love. In fact, Melissa found it hard to take her father as a father and she actually admitted that she needed a partner in him more than a father. The father was valued and longed for, but he was not seen as a father, to which his representative reacted completely automatically. Such processes show that in the course of constellation, we not only have access to knowledge about other people, but we are also governed by certain overriding dynamics, which in a way tells the representatives what is right.

When, after constellation sessions, I ask the clients how they feel, they usually answer in the same way: "More complete." This universal feeling is also unique and is rather not experienced in everyday life. Generally, in constellations, feelings—of both the representatives and the client—can change immediately when the system situation alters, for example, when someone who was excluded appears in the constellation. This is unexpected and informative—it shows that emotions are not primary, but depend on the system constellation.

THE CONSTELLATION THERAPIST'S WORK

Initial Interview

What is the role of the therapist in systemic constellations, what should he do, and what must he avoid? Hellinger stresses the importance of the phenomenological approach. According to this approach, the therapist observes the phenomena arising during therapy, limiting his interventions and interpretations. The therapist can position another representative, ask two people to look at each other, ask someone who lies with the deceased to stand up, and so on. However, he always gives space and time to the developing process and never assumes in advance which direction it will go. To be able to work this way, he must get rid of his previous ideas, expectations, assessments, and hasty conclusions. Also, he should not have a strong intention to help, to change the individual, or his environment, because this way he could easily overlook what really happens and follow his own expectations. Obviously, the therapist is more active when facilitating individual constellations in which he does not use help from the group. In this case, the therapist represents each person and at the same time uses his intuition and rational thinking to plan the next steps of the constellation.

Before the constellation, I usually conduct an initial interview. Sometimes it is short and limited to the client's articulation of the problem; sometimes it is extensive. I can also ask additional questions during the constellation, for instance, about the grandparents, birth circumstances, and siblings. When the client tells me his story, as recommended by Hellinger, I refrain from identifying with his point of view and look at the whole of his family, and those who he does not consider important enough. Keeping this in mind is especially important in instances where we instinctively advocate one of the parties, for instance, when the client talks about rape, incest, brutality of one of the parents. In this case, if the therapist assumes the client's perspective, that is, negatively evaluates one of the persons, he will not be able to help him. The therapist should rather, for the sake of balance, take the side of the excluded, perpetrators of evil, demonized, or ignored persons. Only then will he be ready to show the wider context of the client's situation, and only this can have a truly healing effect.

While talking to the client, I remain aware that I am in touch with the client's field. It is felt psychophysically and provides specific clues. It happens that as soon as the client sits down and starts talking about himself, I have to interrupt him, feeling great tension. I cannot talk anymore, I have to start the constellation immediately because I could not focus anyway. Such situations take place when there is something particularly heavy in the client's system, which is just below the surface and wants to be displayed. At other times, when I want to move to the constellation after the initial conversation, something blocks me. Sometimes I have the impression that it is only me that wants to work, while the client and his system say, "Not yet." It is a sign for me that something important has not been said yet. In this situation, I tell the client about my blockade and ask what may still be important. Sometimes the problem is reformulated because another matter comes to the fore.

Hellinger refers to the emotional attunement to the client's entire system as systemic empathy. Although one can have certain insights into the client's situation as early as during the initial interview (which is related to the focus on the knowing field), the facilitator should refrain from suggesting solutions in this phase. The strength of constellations is precisely that they go beyond our ability for insight. What is the most important in the systemic constellation work is the constellation process, not presumptions or—even if they are correct—the therapist's interpretations. Consistency and adequacy of the constellation surpasses any verbal descriptions of the client's problem.

During the conversation, I treat the client with respect, and I am open to his experiences and point of view. Often, the clients give various explanations for their difficulties, talking about, for example, their overprotective mother, alcoholic father, or quarrels in the family. The therapist knows from experience that the real causes of problems go beyond these patterns. However, he does not try to "convert" the client and show him that this is not the way. This is what the constellation is for.

I often see dysfunctional elements of the client's personality—inadequate emotions and attitudes, or bizarre views about the loved ones. Sometimes I comment on it, but I treat these comments only as a kind of "warm-up," I never want the client to try to change as a result of my comment. As Hellingerian therapists, we are in this privileged situation that during a conversation we do not have to understand much, we can turn, with ignorance and curiosity, to what exists outside the client-therapist relationship, to the knowledge contained in the family field. Therefore, we do not have to demand too much from the client's words, and he does not have to put all his hope in us. In some natural way, we maintain a proper distance from the client's life.

At one of the group workshops, the client, Amelia, could not formulate her problem. She behaved as if she expected me or the group to find it for her. She said that she "had a lot of problems," that she "definitely had a problem," but there was nothing that she was really determined to work on. She referred to another person from the group who had suggested that she have a constellation, implying that maybe she could say something about her problems. She talked mainly about her bad relationship with the mother-in-law, but one did not feel her real determination to work on this issue either. I felt increasing anger, and I have this feeling extremely seldom when talking to clients. I told Amelia that I could not see what we could work on at the moment, and said to the group that "it is good when a client has a problem because it is the plane where we can meet and start working." I suggested to Amelia—meeting her expectations in a way—that she definitely had a problem with her mother. She replied that it could be true because her mother was "not perfect" and that we could work on it. However, I did not feel she really wanted to. When I asked her additional questions, she finally said that basically the present relationship with her mother suited her.

Surely there are therapists who would refuse to facilitate a constellation for this client, claiming she is not motivated or not ready for it. However, I always try to give something to the client, assuming that if he came, he must expect something. I decided to facilitate the only possible constellation at that moment—I brought in a representative of the client and of "something/someone that is her problem." The representative of the client did not want to look at the "problem." They walked around, the "problem" walked out the door, and finally sat on the floor. The representative of the client was angry all that time. It was not a surprise to me, but I supposed it was not her anger or it was inadequate anger. I added a representative I defined as "someone who is related to it."

It changed the situation completely. The new person lay down on the floor, and the "problem" sat down next to her. The representative of the client was cold, she wanted someone to embrace her. I added Amelia's mother. In my opinion, the constellation showed that there was something important in the family that the client unconsciously perceived in her childhood. Something that she was angry about as a child. It was a child's judgment based on partial perception and knowledge. The solution was to move away from it, leave these matters in the past. Then she could grow up and focus on her life. Observing the constellation, the client said that anger had always been closest to her, that it was the feeling she had known best since childhood. The statement was interesting because in her words or behavior there was not even a trace of anger (of course, this anger flowed in an invisible way, "infecting" me and other people who listened to Amelia, for instance).

Beyond Judgment

The example given above showed that the therapist should not let himself to judge the client and follow his—as it can be called—countertransference. The constellation made it clear that neither unawareness of the problem or inducing anger in the listener was a manifestation of the client's bad will, but was directly rooted in her unconscious attitude and systemic situation.

This is probably how it always is. I remember a workshop in which there was a very obese person. When it was her turn to have a constellation—she came up laughing, irritating by her lack of seriousness. The constellation displayed that she was strongly identified with her grandfather and grandmother who had died in a concentration camp, as well as with the perpetrators. It was such a traumatic event that she had to separate herself from it by her lack of seriousness and her fatness.

When we study different therapeutic methods, we notice that they often contain elements that can cause the client to be judged. Of course, everyone agrees that the therapist is supposed to avoid assessments, but a kind of evaluation is present in therapeutic methods to varying degrees. For example, in psychodynamic therapy, this immanent tendency to evaluate results from a focus on the patient's problems. Treatment consists in identifying and working through conflicts, deficits, and difficulties that are revealed during the interview, through free associations and the therapeutic relationship. The psychodynamic method refers to primitive (primary) defense mechanisms, immature ego, envy, and so on. These terms alone build a specific attitude toward the patient. It is different in systemic constellations. They show a wider context of the functioning of the psyche and direct the therapist toward the areas that are more important than the dynamics of character.

It seems that many therapists drift toward judgment: either the patient is "guilty" because he resists, uses passive aggression, denial and "attacks" interpretations, or other people, generally his parents, are "guilty." It is not direct looking for the guilty ones or judging directly—it would not be psychotherapy at all—but a given mental attitude and methodological approach.

In constellations, we do not speak of the "guilty." During constellations, everything we encounter is embedded into the wider context. The causes have their causes. Though by no means endlessly, as we usually find something that can be considered the primary cause. This is often a random event, such as the death of a newborn child, war, adoption, or difficult labor. Problems and someone's negative behavior start with love and loyalty, for example, when they internally follow their beloved departed or want to compensate for some harm from the distant past. This is why he is unavailable to his own child or aggressive. Could this be judged?

In constellations, regardless of our impression of the client, we do not attach much importance to his personality and way of being, without looking for the essential things in these surface manifestations. For example, a client says that her problem is her contact with the son (an adult who has a partner and lives separately) because he does not spend enough time with her, he prefers other people, and she does not feel confident in his presence. It is very easy to enter into a polemic with her, because it is clearly felt that she wants her son to be a substitute for her partner. However, during the constellation, it turns out that the mother basically did not see her son—she was internally focused on his father, whom she left just after the boy was born. Whereas the son felt a great need for deeper contact with her and only after moving toward her could he turn to his father. The father's first partner (with whom he had a child) also played an important role here. So, although on some level the mother was possessive, she did not accept her son's independence and wanted him to fill her emotional needs, following these matters would not have led us to a solution. It lay somewhere else—as usual beyond what we can capture with a "linear" mind during a conversation.

In traditional therapies, many years of self-therapy and supervision are needed to be able to maintain an undisturbed attitude to the patient. Because the therapeutic process is based on the relationship, the therapist is forced to more or less accept the patient's mental intrusions or transferential demands. This often causes his emotional reactions such as tiredness, reluctance, suppressed anger, or excitement, which we define as countertransferential. Since every patient is different, the therapist in a transference situation must constantly make a new effort to understand and cope. However, due to the fact that in constellations, we use an autonomous and teleological process that leads both the client and the therapist, they can meet beyond transference and countertransference. In constellations, the procedures are so clear and well defined that it is much easier for the therapist to keep an undisturbed attitude, which is constructive for the client. Simply put, if the therapist does not know what is happening, or feels that he is not quite able to deal with emotions, he can withdraw as much as possible, let the representatives act. On the other hand, in individual therapy, as soon as he enters the field of the client's system, his earlier feelings will quickly blur.

The Therapist and the Client's Parents

Hellinger emphasizes that in systemic therapy, the phenomenon of transference and countertransference should not take place, so the relationship must not take the parent-child form. If the facilitator sees not only the client but also his family, respects them, then transference will not occur, and the client's feelings will somehow flow through the therapist to his parents. Also, the therapist must not get involved in the disputes that arise from countertransference or attempts to "fix" the client. He is not allowed to be driven by irritation or anger that his clients' certain attitudes may cause. He must always remember that his function is service-oriented and he should do as much as possible for every client, regardless of whether he feels comfortable with a given person. Another thing is that by bringing about the orders of love, the facilitator's potential irritation also disappears.

Psychotherapy is based on the fact that there are certain causes of every human problem. Many psychotherapeutic schools see these causes in childhood, and this may lead to blaming the patient's parents for his difficulties. It may be tempting to see oneself as a "better parent" and the therapy process as mothering or replacing the father. Such an attitude should be regarded as destructive to the patient's development.

When you listen to conversations of therapists representing various schools, you can sometimes hear an accusatory tone toward the patient's parents. There are phrases like "alcoholic daddy" or "overprotective mummy." By using such words, one belittles the importance of parenting and closes his eyes to the fact that they are the only real parents of the given person. The one who talks this way shows his immaturity. Behind the phrases that depreciate the parents, a child is hidden. He expects "real" and "perfect" parents. The therapist despises the patient's parents because he has not grown to the fact that also his parents are simply human. He never transgressed his infantility and still unconsciously fantasizes about ideal parents. The father or mother may seem "possessive," "cold," "controlling," and finally "inadequate" or "aggressive," which causes the therapist to want to oppose them or instruct them for the good of the patient.

In systemic constellations, we avoid this. It is easier for us because we see parents as no different from our clients. It may seem obvious that no therapist using another therapeutic method will deny that parents are "no different," but experience shows that when he meets the patient's parents, the therapist may become tense, less understanding, more accusing. Working with constellations, we perceive the parents as the people who, just like the client, have their parents and are their children. They have their own burdens and are not the "source" of their child's problems.

The therapists who do not fully know the strength of the bond may have the impression that through their understanding, accepting, calm, sympathetic, attentive, or any other attitude they give the patient what his parents did not give him. Such thinking is wrong. Even if the mother did not notice the child's needs, she was cold and emotionally absent, what she gave the child, that is, life, outweighs the therapist's gift many times. It is similar with the father.

Systemic constellations do not create substitutes or illusions here. They provide an opportunity to find the real parents and to not mistake the therapist for them. The clear approach to this issue makes an unambiguous formation of the therapist possible. He stops competing with the client's parents as well as judging them or trying to replace them. In constellations, we work with the client's actual parents, of whom the therapist (or workshop participant) becomes a representative. He is then a kind of gateway to the parent, which leads very far in the therapeutic process. It is also safer for the client, as opposed to situations where the therapist becomes a transferential or surrogate parent.

From the Last and Last But One Row

Hellinger says that the constellation therapist helps "from the last row." This attitude does not result from the innate modesty of systemic therapists, but from the fact that constellations make this style of work possible, and thanks to it, we can achieve maximum effects. In constellations, what is most important happens without anyone's guidance. In many correctly facilitated constellations, the therapist is not much more than an organizer, enabling reality that is beyond his consciousness and intention, as well as beyond the consciousness of the client, manifest itself. The essential elements of the constellation can appear and be solved spontaneously, or they can be proposed by the representatives, captivated by the system and its orders. So the therapist does not have anything that is inaccessible to other workshop participants. If the constellation is done with the help of representatives, they have a decisive role in it, and their feelings and systemic intuitions can go beyond what the therapist sees.

It is a little different during individual constellations. Here the therapist helps from the last but one row, because more depends on him. He has to think "what to do next"—who else to bring in the constellation, on which position to stand now, when to ask the client what he feels and what to draw his attention to, how long to stay in a given role, what sentences of strength to propose to the client, when to finish the constellation. Despite the fact that on a certain level, the therapist controls the course of the constellation, on another one, he fully surrenders to what is happening. I define it as work from a double perspective.

In systemic constellations, it is easier than in other therapeutic methods to keep an ethical and service-oriented attitude toward clients. It is easier to not get involved in arguments with clients, to not abuse one's position, and to remain a professional who only "does his job." Both the client and the therapist wait for something that will only surface during the constellation process. What is manifested is independent of the therapist and often requires no comment from him, being understood by the client without any explanation. Therefore, clients do not focus on the therapist. In other methods, the therapist's personality often determines the shape of the meeting. The constellation therapist disappears behind the technique and what is displayed. In no case should he see himself as a guru, a person that "radiates with love" or someone particularly sensitive. Facilitating constellations is, in this respect, available to most averagely sensitive people. The processes—hitherto considered unusual—are treated in constellations as ordinary tools that can be used by any properly trained and experienced person.

WORKING ON THE CLIENT'S INNER ATTITUDE

Unconscious Attitudes

In constellations, we work with the system and the client's inner world, that is, with his inner attitude. Working classically or individually, we pay attention to what happens to the client during the constellation and actively try to help him change what is unconstructive in his inner world. Originally, Hellinger paid a lot of attention to the client's inner attitude. He frequently required that the sentence be repeated if the client did not speak it with conviction. Therefore, he actively supported the presence of the client in the constellation process.

Constellations show that the inner and generally unconscious attitude can be different from the outer one. Someone verbally rejects his father, while internally he turns to him. Someone else declares attachment and respect for the mother, and internally has great difficulty in bowing to her. Sometimes it is difficult for the client to express and acknowledge something, the acknowledgment of which would seem obvious. For example, he cannot say to his parents, "You are my parents." What is not a problem when filling the "Parents" section in documents becomes impossible here. It is bringing to light the hidden attitude toward the parents, sometimes surprising to the client himself, but usually quickly felt as true (obviously this difficulty does not result from the fact that the representative is not the real father or mother, but because during the constellation, there is a confrontation with the deep, not surface attitude toward the parents).

Standing in front of the client—for example, as his father—I am not only in the role, which means that I react as the person from his system, I also remain the therapist and observe the client's reactions. I ask how he feels, if something is changing within him. I also insert a "probe" into his mind. I try to empathize with his attitude "from the inside." It can be said that I am in three modes at the time: I feel as a representative, think like a therapist, and perceive the client's feelings. I do it especially when there is a problem, a blockage. For example, the client says that he cannot fully accept his father (whom I represent), that something is blocking him. I try to get to know the problem better, sense what is happening. To do it, I also try to mentally, without abandoning the role of the father, feel the client's attitude. I would describe it as a pulsating movement in which I alternately have feelings of the father and the son. During such probing, I can come to the conclusion that the client is afraid of something, that he is angry, or that it is difficult for him to give up his own uniqueness and the like. I can notice that he is like a small child who imagined that so much depends on him, I can feel the weight he carries in himself, sense the difficulty in his going to his life, or the desire to cling to his parents.

A constellation makes it possible to uncover emotions and attitudes that we suppress and which we do not want to admit to ourselves. Jacqueline suffered from back pains since early youth, and they got worse recently. She also had other diseases, such as thyroid problems and rheumatism, which she described as "autoaggressive." I asked her to stand in the middle of the room and choose a representative of her spine. The representative felt something in her own spine and lay down on the floor. I also entered the constellation as "something/someone else that also mattered here." I lay down spontaneously next to the spine. In the further course of the work, there were the following representations: "other diseases," "anger," and "someone Jacqueline was most angry with." Jacqueline's anger appeared when I joined as "something/someone else that also mattered here." The client started pushing me, and I was backing away.

Then we started working with her inner states. The client did not immediately contact her anger and did not recognize its strength. She only said that I made her angry. However, when I moved away from her, I could look into her inner world and see the extraordinary scale of her anger. That is why I suggested the sentences that could express this:

T: "I'm angry with you."
C: Yes, I'm angry with you.
T: "I'm furious."
C: Yes, but I must suppress it, I can't show it. This is constant suppression.
T: There's even more here: "I could kill you."
C: Yes, I could kill you. And what am I supposed to do with it? I must be paralyzed.

She said that she wanted to hit me in the stomach and to "smash in" another representative's head. When the representative of "someone Jacqueline was most angry with" approached her, she felt downright murderous fury. He was not afraid of her, however, and Jacqueline did not like it at all.

When I stood next to her, I realized that she imagined that she was a monster and that she could frighten any man (by the way, she did not care about her appearance).

It was an insight related to simultaneous being in the client's field and the system's field. I shared it, adding sarcastically: "Godzilla has come, that's how you imagine yourself." I also said, "Maybe it's time to leave those dreams that you're a monster and scare everyone? Maybe you're just an ordinary girl?" Then Jacqueline said as if she had a brainwave: "I know. I know who first said I was the devil—grandpa." She had a lot of negative feelings for her grandfather, which resulted from the fact that he treated her and her mother badly. I suggested that Jacqueline say to him, "I leave it with you, grandpa." I also asked her to accept the dead grandfather as a "soul," without his words or deeds.

Jacqueline had many constellations, but she considered this work to be the key one, stating that it was an important work on the "structures of the subject." Her back pain disclosed her disrespect and lack of obeisance (not only toward the grandfather) and suppressed enormous anger—generalized and felt toward many people, but rooted in her relationship with the grandfather.

For Bettina, it was right to say to her grandfather, who died when she was six (and who had some family secrets): "Dear grandfather, you have a place in my heart, you still live there. I am only a child, only a granddaughter, I'm leaving everything that is not mine." Bettina took her beloved grandfather's death very hard, and the memory of him still aroused strong emotions in her. However, it was difficult for her to utter those words. So I asked her to simply say, "I accept you as my grandfather." She replied, "Yes, I accept you, I have always accepted you." When the client says that something has always been or that he has known it all for a long time, it is a red flag for the therapist. I asked her twice if she really accepted her grandfather. Then the client shouted, "No, I don't accept him! I'm angry that he left me."

It was a typical phenomenon—a child's anger with a loved one for having passed away. I deduced from this that Bettina was, in part, still the six-year-old child. This state was due to her anger with her grandfather, the difficulty in looking at him and in accepting him. Now the moment came when she was supposed to leave her infantile attitude and accept the grandfather. She would gain strength, her fear of death would be reduced, and she could take her life in her own hands. However, Bettina replied, "No, no. I don't want to, I could only be a child with him. I've always been an adult." So it became clear to me that I had to lead her the opposite way. I asked her to sit even closer to her grandfather and say, "I remain a child, with you, grandpa." It was only this that gave her relief. Did I abandon my original goal, which was to lead the client to maturity? Of course not. But her step in this direction, the one she was ready for, was just that—to express the bond with her grandfather and her childlike part. Both of these things were hidden, as was her anger that covered them.

Inner Parentification

I asked Eveline to choose a figurine to represent her. "But an adult or a child one?"—she asked and chose a child figurine. At my request, she also set up her mother and father, followed by her grandmother and sister. In the further part of the constellation, the mother's aborted child appeared too. At the beginning, the parents stood on both sides of Eveline, as in a pincer movement. However, she felt fine. When I slowly turned her figurine to face the mother, the client said it was a strange feeling, something surprising and unusual. After a while she said that it is difficult for her to look at herself as a child and that, in some moments, she wanted to set up an adult figurine. I suggested the words, "Mom, I'm your child." Eveline could not say that, but said that the word "big" came to her mind. "I'm big, not adult, but big." I suggested that she say, "Mom, I'm your little child, only a child." When

Eveline wanted to say it, the word "big" stood in the way. Then I said that one can be a child or an adult who contains that child, but there is no such person as a "big one."

After some time, Eveline began to feel that she could be a child. Now it was clear how much she needed from her mother. At the end, I exchanged her figurine into an adult one, saying that as an adult she could take too. After the constellation, Eveline was still thinking about the word "big." She said she had never thought of herself that way before, but during the session she felt it clearly.

Eveline could not live an adult and independent life—she could not finish anything, she had an apartment and a partner, but she could not stop living with her parents, she kept failing her profession admission exam. In her childhood, she was very independent, as many children who cannot cope in adulthood. Now Eveline was "big," but not adult. She could not become adult because there was a child in her who was still hungry for the mother. This child could not be satiated, as Eveline was "big" and one can take from the mother only from the position of a child.

The way to solve this problem could not be to try to become an adult, but to recognize her childlike needs, and thus to accept the hierarchy, and the mother as a mother. It is only after this act that the process of becoming a true adult begins. One can only grow up if one does not skip the child's stage.

"Resistance" in Constellations

In constellations, the therapist, the representatives, and the client himself follow the orders of love, and the therapy is immersed in an objective, external process. This causes that we do not have to convince the client of anything, because basically he sees the same as the therapist. We also do not have to offer gains that will come later in exchange for the painfulness of the therapy, because the session leads toward positive emotions that can be felt immediately. Despite this, it happens that the client resists to accept the solution. Usually, however, resistance is not permanent and is overcome during a constellation. Resistance may result from the following:

- The solution evokes a sense of guilt for transgressing the unwritten laws of the family;
- Being sick gives a sense of innocence and belonging, and health and solving the problem makes one lonely;
- Resigning from the symbiotic relationship (entanglement) and entering into the "face-to-face" relationship are associated with a moment of separation and loneliness;

- Giving back what burdened us may be associated with a temporary sense of emptiness;
- Leaving a parent or other person to their own emotions and fate may cause pain and the desire to go back to the original attitude;
- Carrying the affairs of the older members of the system and violating the hierarchy may give a sense of being someone special;
- Giving up the familiar, even destructive, way of life may be related to the fear of stepping into the unknown;
- Following the archaic sense of justice or the need for atonement is sometimes strong and difficult to change;
- In case of the interrupted movement toward the mother or father, it may take a longer time to restore the original feelings.

The client who resists usually sees where the solution lies and partly agrees that it may be good for him. It is just that something stands in his way and is beyond his control at the moment. In such cases, he usually follows some loyalty or inner sense of justice. For example, he cannot solve his problems, because it would mean that he would stop demanding compensation for the harm done to him by his parents.

The client's resistance does not result from his bad will. It is often an indication that we have not considered something or are doing something too quickly (Franke 2003, 80). In this case, it may be difficult for the client to say sentences of strength, accept his parents, leave something in the past, and so on. This type of resistance is justified and informs the therapist that the constellation is not complete. One of the basic indicators of the therapist's competency level is the ability to notice the information that comes from resistance. The therapist who treats resistance solely as the client's personal problem still needs to learn a lot. The client is not able to fully accept the solution, because his fixed attitude stands in the way, but when we add something in the constellation, we will make its change possible.

Mark could not leave with his mother the burden that he unconsciously took on himself as a child. It was his mother's emotional states, whose roots lay in an even deeper past. Obviously, he was not aware of these things, and it was only the constellation that brought them to light. It addressed his obesity and showed that he in a way "fed" himself with what he took.

Mark felt that if he left this burden, he would be completely "empty" and his mother would become "alien" to him. He had the impression that without the burdens that had shaped him since childhood, he would lose his identity, almost cease to exist, which aroused his fear and caused resistance. However, when I asked the mother to turn to the earlier generations and leave what she had taken (I had the impression that she had taken it with nonchalance, in a way flirted with it in her life, then fed her son with it), Mark got the opportunity to leave the weight with her. Why were these processes connected? When the mother left what belonged to the past generations, the son could finally feel her as a mother. She came out from behind the curtain of burdens that had covered her until now. Having a mother, Mark could "fill up" with her, not with what came from the past.

An interesting phenomenon is one's difficulty in accepting the discovery that the parent's complaints or excessive expectations that hurt the client, in fact, did not concern him at all, because they were transferred from another relationship. It seems that such insight should only unburden, and yet a sense of losing one's meaning may occur. Carina's mother kept repeating that she had wasted her daughter's life. She said, "If I were a better mother, it would be different." The daughter felt really burdened with these words, all the more she did not consider her life a failure. The constellation showed that the mother did not accept the death of her older son. She accused herself, believed she could have done something to prevent it. Saying that if she had acted differently, her daughter's life would be better, she was in fact referring to her deceased son. The truth was too painful, and the son was taboo. Another thing was that she turned away from her son by rejecting the true fate. Therefore, he was never mourned, and his death was not part of the narrative of the family. When Carina understood this, at first she felt disappointed that her mother did not mean her.

Resistance may result from guilt. Malvina blamed herself for allowing surgery on her few-year-old daughter, who lost her eye as a result. The chances to save it were minimal, and if the surgery had not been performed, the daughter could have died. Still, Malvina seemed to regret her decision and wanted to turn back time. During the constellation, it was clear how the daughter needed her mother to just be there for her—like every child she wanted a strong mother in her maternal role. However, Malvina seemed to blame herself persistently and did not consider herself a good enough mother. Eventually, it took the form of rejecting the daughter. The daughter wanted her as a mother, but she did not fully accept herself as a mother. In this way, she deprived her daughter of a mother.

Sometimes resistance arises from a lack of readiness to change one's perception of the family system. This may be the case for young people who are still dependent on their parents. They may have grudges against their parents, expect them to change, and at the same time not want to change their opinion about them. They have every right to do so. It is different for adults, who should be ready to change their perspective. Some people, however, fear that changing their view of the family and themselves will result in a loss of belonging.

This was the case with Martha, who adopted the attitude of a little girl that insisted on not changing her view of the family. She seemed to believe that obedience to her mother, and a kind of not acknowledging the relationship with her ex-partner, would guarantee her the status of a child. Her infantilism, a kind of lack of emotions, not taking responsibility for her own problems and a fixed smile made almost everyone in the group feel angry. In the end, the client accepted as much as she could, and in any case, she took a step forward.

The constellation of a thirty-two-year-old Thomas shows what may be the roots of the attitude of not taking responsibility for one's own problems. Thomas complained about depression, difficulties in entering into a relationship with a woman, and the problem of putting the needs of others over his own needs. When we were working on his father's and grandfather's important issues, he asked, "But what does this have to do with me?" He said, "You have to move on," leave the past behind. During the constellation, however, he realized that he had not left the past behind at all, and was repeating the old patterns. Although he had the opportunity to put many things in order, he did not see much sense in it. What was the reason, why did he not want to do anything about it? At some point, I understood it and said, "Now I know what you mean. You feel as if you were told to solve something for others. You would like to say, I apologize for the word: Damn, why should I do that!" Thomas smiled wryly and said, "Well, that's right." He considered the constellation to be another weight and task, and yet it is the adults who should put things in order in the family.

When I worked with Anna, I used figurines. Anna was in a relationship with a priest. It seemed like her figurine was looking at something, so I put a girl figurine as "what she was looking at." Then I asked her to position her parents. They were turned away from each other and felt almost nothing. I asked if there was something difficult happening in the mother's family. It turned out that her older, mentally ill brother had been taken to a care facility and "had gone missing." When he had been still living in his family home, he had always been happy when his sister had come to visit him. I set up the mother's brother, then turned the figurine representing Anna toward her uncle, suggesting the words, "You're my uncle who was sent away to the care facility. I've been really concerned about your fate."

A: But I didn't think about him.
T: "I didn't think about you, but inside I was concerned."
A: Yes.

When she was in primary school, Anna felt that she had to kneel on the pavement, "so that mother would come back," for the same purpose she had to scribble with a pen in her notebook until she made a hole, or kiss the floor in the church. Finally, she was sent to a psychiatrist. I said that maybe her uncle also kneeled so that the mother would come back. Anna moved the figurine of her uncle closer to her figurine. Later, the mother and uncle stood opposite their parents (Anna's grandparents). I had a feeling of harmony, but when I asked Anna how she felt, she replied, "Worse. This here—she pointed to her grandparents, mother and uncle—is so ordinary." So I placed the client's partner in front of her, suggesting she say the words, "I like you also because the relationship with you is strange."—"Yes," she said, looking at the picture for a long time.

However, maybe Anna did not need the extraordinary, but this identification with her uncle caused that she had to have an elusive partner? For the uncle, the beloved mother and sister were elusive too. And the priest was elusive doubly, because in addition, he cheated on her.

Sometimes it may seem that the client's resistance has a rational basis and results from resistance to the method itself, to its extraordinary nature. This was the case with Patrick. He attempted suicide, he suffered from depression, he felt constantly weakened and unable to live independently, and work caused him distress. When I stood as his depression, I saw that someone else in the family was depressed or in mourning. I stood as "what his condition resulted from" and grabbed my neck, I began to spin and wobble. I asked if anyone in the family committed suicide. Patrick did not know anything about it. When I asked him about his feelings, he answered that he did not feel anything, that he was in such a situation for the first time, that it was all strange. He seemed to be cutting himself off from the strange method and the therapist's strange behavior.

Patrick mentioned that his parents "told him about it too," that "it is some kind of shamanism." These and his other words along with the feelings I had during the constellation, helped me understand his attitude. I said, "It's the others who speak through you." I asked him to turn around and imagine his parents opposite him. Then Patrick started to feel. He said that he wanted to leave their patterns with them, that he wanted to finally start thinking independently, that he had a right to do so, that they did not always have to be right. His body was trembling, and he was making movements as if he wanted to throw something off himself. His initial resistance and lack of feeling were directly proportional to his later dramatic attempts to throw off what bound him by unnecessary loyalty to his parents.

THE FUNCTION OF THE DECEASED AND NONPERSONAL ELEMENTS

The Dead and the Living

Basically, the living and the deceased do not differ much in constellations. We approach both in a similar way. However, we can say that there are three "types" of the dead in constellations: the supportive ones, the ones we follow, and the traumatizing ones. Although this probably has nothing to do with their "afterlife." The supporting deceased is, for example, our parent we have taken into the heart, it is the one who "stands behind us" even if he has been dead for many years. The deceased we follow into death is, for example, the father's brother who died in childhood and about whom we did not even know. The traumatizing deceased may be the early deceased mother, the memory of whom is too painful, or the son who committed suicide. Of course, in fact, all the deceased are similar, and there are no friendly or unfriendly ones. It is us who perceive them in different ways. Every deceased can become a supportive deceased, if we give him a place in the heart and at the same time, accept his fate with respect.[1]

However, to be able to fully accept the deceased, sometimes a constellation is needed. During the constellation, we do something not only for ourselves but also for the dead. For instance, we help our deceased parents find their parents. Or we let the victims and perpetrators to join together, even in the fourth generation. Then the restless dead calm down. Is this spiritism? Do we try to manipulate the world of "spirits"? Someone who sees it this way cannot free himself from the patterns of religion. What we can say empirically is that there is a change for the better in the living. We achieve it considering the dead. However, we must take seriously the feelings of relief that occur in the representatives of the dead. Constellations not only reconstruct the past but also modify interpersonal processes and bring about order. This often causes that the dead, who finally gets noticed and accepted, gains peace. Perhaps the deceased is only an aspect of the client's mind, but the easiest way is to say that it is this person who has gained peace.

Alice lost her 20-year-old son in a car accident. Due to adaptive disorder in the form of a depressive response, she visited a psychiatrist and started psychotherapy in my office. She had transient hallucinations, in which she saw her son lying in different places, just as he had been lying at the accident site. In the first constellation, with the use of figurines, the figurines of the living formed a kind of circle, and the figurine of the deceased son looked over their shoulder. It was clearly isolated.

After a few months of therapy, Alice started the next session by telling me that she felt her son intensely again. I asked her to write his name on a piece of paper. It was difficult for her to do it, she felt blocked, said she did not like it when someone pronounced his name or even when it was mentioned in movies. Eventually, she wrote her son's name and put the piece of paper about a meter away. I asked the client how she felt. She answered that she could hear her son's voice as if from a distance, and that she did not understand what he was saying. When I stood in the son's place, I felt that he was turning toward his mother, expecting to be accepted, noticed. I asked Alice how she felt about her son. She said she felt nothing, because it was not him. Of course, one could agree with her if we did not know how constellations work. Then the patient said that her son was calling her over. At that moment I felt extremely weak—the mother's attitude was making her son break down. I said that he was not calling her over, that he wanted her to stay where she was. He also wanted her to see where he was. I said, as the son, "Why don't you look at me?" The client replied, "Because you're gone." Then she added that she felt as if she had been standing over the grave.

The client was unable to grant her son—as a departed—a place in her heart. Hence her prolonged mourning, or rather depression with psychotic symptoms (I leave aside the other factors that shaped Alice into a person susceptible to this type of condition). I suggested the following sentence: "I can't take you into my heart, because that would mean grieving," but the client could not say it. She kept her son in a kind of transition space—he was neither alive nor dead.

Here, we come to an interesting conclusion, which is supported by constellations with other people. In order to be able to deal with mourning, we must first recognize that the deceased is not among the living, so it is not him who appears on the street and calls us. Second, recognizing his existence in "another reality" helps us. It seems to be healthy and natural for a person to recognize that "in some way" his beloved deceased still exists. Fierce disbelief seems to be connected with pathological conditions such as depression. I do not mean faith in the religious sense. The fact that the deceased "exist" is supported by facts—how else could we see their fate and reactions in constellations or make reconciliation with the deceased parents possible?

In the constellation described above, it was important for the mother to see "where the son was." What did this mean? She was to consider him dead and existing at the same time. Although it looks like a paradox, there may be no other way to deal with pathological mourning. Only when we see the dead as "existing" can we admit full awareness that he is dead. Otherwise, his death will be internally denied, and he will return in the form of pathological projections such as auditory hallucinations. The mother was aware of her son's death and yet did not accept it, still hearing him. But why did she hear him, claiming at the same time that he was "gone"? It was precisely for the above reasons.

Nonpersonal Elements

In constellations, we assign also abstract and nonpersonal roles to representatives. These may be "fate," "death," "support," "illness," "birth," "work," or "money." What is the function and meaning of such elements? What does it mean that the house the client is trying to sell "feels better" in a given arrangement? Can inanimate objects have their own attitudes or feelings and want something? And what is "death" or "fate" in a constellation?

When we bring in nonpersonal elements in constellations, most of them transform and indicate specific people. For example, an illness may represent a person to whom someone is unconsciously bound. Money may "turn out to be" the client's mother—it is just that his attitude toward his mother is what determines his money-related problems most. If something like money appears in a constellation, it is not money in general, but the client's "internal" money—his attitude to money, his financial history.

However, some abstract representations do not relate to persons, but have meaning themselves. These are "death" and "life," for example. When someone positions himself, "death" and "life," his individual dynamics toward these existentially important realities will manifest itself. Someone will turn away from "life" and head toward "death." Someone else will want to coerce "death" into something, for example, to move it further away from himself. The representative of someone's life will feel extremely weak, and the representative of someone else's life will wait in vain for them to get closer. What do we actually work with in such constellations? With the deep levels of the client's mind, with his attitude to his own life, and to death, which is an inseparable part of this life. All this translates into the functioning of the given person, his health or ability to achieve goals.

Judith had a lot of paralyzing concerns and anxieties about the lives of her loved ones. One could say that she saw death everywhere. She said, however, "I'm not afraid of death, I can die." We sometimes say that someone has "contempt" for death. What does it result in? It puts the individual in a delusional position that weakens his true capabilities, sometimes causes anxiety. In the constellation, I asked Judith to bow down before "death," before its greatness and independence. Then "death" felt it could take a step back. As long as Judith did not recognize its domination, "death" was close all the time. That is why she saw it everywhere.

Not all nonpersonal objects that appear in constellations have the same status. Roles such as "death" and "life" have a stronger ontic status than the "*alter ego*" or "happiness." An important element of many constellations is "fate." Not as a personification of destiny, but a kind of synthesis of a wide range of factors that affected the fate of the family, parents, and the client himself. The function of the representative of fate is clearly visible, for example, when a child is unable to accept his parent because of a great grievance and accusations. It may concern an emotionally absent, indifferent parent, or an alcoholic. Even if he sees the entanglement of his father or mother, for example, the fact that they have followed the deceased internally all their lives, the client is unable to forgive them. He is still treating them as the only creators of their own lives and his life. However, when we show "fate" to such a child, positioning it behind his parent, his feelings change. Then the therapist's words that the parent "did not decide about everything" start to finally make sense to him. The client becomes aware of the perspective in which his own life takes place and his fate is shaped. Thus, he goes beyond the narrow picture of a "child harmed by his evil parents." He becomes calm and accepting. When he sees "fate" as something separate from the parent, he becomes able to accept the father or the mother. Such a constellation illustrates well the power of personification and its healing potential. It is only by looking at one's "fate," that in the constellation has the face of the representative, that makes the client able to understand and change his inner attitude.

The representation of war has a similar function; it indicates a supraindividual force that influenced relationships in the family over generations. This force was beyond the control of anyone in the family, but everyone felt its effects. "War" is not an abstraction, and bringing it in the constellation is not a purely technical procedure. This is an indication of a real factor that at certain times governed the fate of millions of people.

Strangely enough, however, within the family, it is not clearly noticed. The family members tend to look at one another and their relationships without seeing this powerful causative factor. The children and grandchildren, even if they know that their father or grandmother survived a concentration camp, lost their parents or children, or experienced something terrible as soldiers, look at the family relationships and behaviors of their parents or grandparents without taking these events into account. The attitude of all those involved in these events, who do not talk about their experiences at all or talk about them in a simplistic and shallow way, usually strengthens this kind of perception. In the end, the impact of war and its determining character becomes, as it were, repressed. However, its negative emotional consequences persist in the family. In a constellation, by showing war as a very important factor, we bring about the right perspective and enable emotions and relationships to be healed.

SYSTEMIC CONSTELLATIONS AS A METHOD OF COGNITION

Cognition in Constellations

My field of perception and reflection in systemic constellations is wide. First of all, through representation, I get information about the people important to the client and about their relationships. Second, I receive feedback from the client. It is not only memories but also current experiences and completely new insights and hitherto forgotten information that emerge as a result of the constellation. Third, I can approach the client's inner attitude through empathizing. Fourth, I directly feel the adequacy of the suggested sentences and the order that has been brought about. For instance, when I stand as the client's father, and the client says that he leaves what is not his with me, I immediately feel a surge of strength—if he actually does this internally. When he is unable to give back the burden or he subconsciously keeps holding a grudge against his parent—I spontaneously move away.

The knowledge of the client's situation acquired through constellations is accurate—it contains important components of his family relationships, internal state, and sometimes also health problems. An example would be the individual session with Malcolm. He felt pain in his right side. I stood as the "cause" of the pain. In this role, I shook my right arm, which was somehow weakened, a bit inert, I felt as if there was "something traumatic" in this arm. Malcolm said that when he was 14 years old, he fell from a tree onto his right arm, he could not straighten it out, now he had two metal rods in his shoulder. They should have been removed, but they were not.

Therapist: Why?
Client: My mother neglected it.
T: Do you have a grudge against your mother?
C: I think so.

I stood as the mother, I gestured over the "cause" sheet as if I wanted to form a dome, soothe something, and silence it. The client said that his mother constantly worried about him (his twin brother had died before, which was the subject of our previous work). I said it looked like the mother did not want to look at something, like she wanted to have peace.

Client: That's how it was, mother gave me apples and locked me in the room so that I would sit quietly.

At some point, the client's aunt, his mother's sister, who had a big influence on the mother, came to his mind. I stood as that aunt, and immediately felt I wanted to push the client away from his mother. I felt tensed and nervous. I told the client about it and said that this tension was connected to the aunt's personal history. The client confirmed, "Yes, my aunt is nervous all the time." After a while, he said that his aunt said that she liked him and other similar things. I had this thought too, about something erotic on the part of the aunt, but I refrained from saying this.

The client mentioned his father, so I brought him in the constellation. At some point, he had fights with his father, and attended karate classes because he wanted to defend his mother. The father had trained in boxing before. As the father, I approached the son and simulated a series of boxing punches on his chest. Although he had mentioned martial arts before, these moves were by no means deliberate, they appeared spontaneously. Malcolm said that he felt threatened when I approached him. As the father, I felt I was rather having fun than being aggressive. There was something infantile about it, as if I treated the son like a friend, and did not see I was a father, whereas the son took it seriously and was paralyzed by fear. I turned 180 degrees and imagined that I was standing in front of my own father (Malcolm's grandfather). I immediately felt that Malcolm's father had difficulty accepting his father. After a while, it turned out that his mother too, as I imagined her standing in front of me. The client said that his father's parents had died early—this explained the disruption of the bond with them.

In the constellation, I could clearly see—and could indirectly feel—the whole complex of fears of the client. In fact, I had access to the states of his "inner child." I saw the anxiety about the mother who was beaten by the father, the anxiety taken over from the mother caused by the death of her children, the confusion about the aunt's attitude, the fear of her anger, the fear of the father, and the trauma associated with his hand physical injury.

Cognitive Machine

When the traditional therapist listens to the patient, he may wonder how his functioning has been influenced by the patterns built up in his childhood, compare his attitude to that of his father or mother, and try to discover the relationship between his current functioning and the childhood events or other facts. These attempts may not provide enough knowledge to solve the patient's problems. The therapist's projections and premature conclusions, which are only seemingly correct, are an obstacle. The most important limitation is that the therapist is not able to process the mass of information reaching him. The patient constantly consciously and unconsciously communicates something, but ordering it is beyond the analytical abilities of the mind. Therefore, even if the therapist has empathy, intuition, and reads the patient's unconscious messages, he will still not be able to grasp all the dependencies of his problem.

Systemic constellations provide a whole new quality here. They not only reveal information about the client's situation but also make it easier to analyze and infer. They work in a similar way to a sheet of paper when calculating—it is obvious that complicated calculations cannot be carried out in memory. Constellations are a "machine" that enables to relieve the therapist's mind. The use of space is essential here. When, instead of just thinking about relationships, we present them in space, we let the information condense, and we have easy access to it. As one physicist said, space is "data compression on a massive scale" (in: Musser 2015, 177). Constellations have something of a tactic board, on which representations of military units are placed, then moved and reorganized. Spatial visualization helps to encompass the situation and think.[2]

Another important element is constellation sequentiality. We can see it well in a constellation with figurines or sheets of paper, where each successive step results from the previous ones. We do not immediately see the whole and move to the solution, but follow the sequence of events. At a given moment, we deal with the feelings and movement of the mother, then the father, the deceased child, and someone from the past. When working with figurines, each change in the position of a given figurine has an impact on the further course of the constellation and brings us closer to the final image. This final image is not predictable, but is the result of the subsequent, interrelated stages. In this layer, a constellation resembles the work of a Turing machine (computer), where the result comes from certain subsequent steps. This relieves the mind, as we concentrate on the sequence and do not speedily look for a solution.

In a constellation, we can represent the relevant people, not just think about them. This means that the therapist does not have to "simulate" them all in his consciousness, recall the facts related to them, and consider their mutual relations. Such a method would lead to simplifications and distortions. Instead, he "checks" what "is happening to the mother," "how the grandmother is feeling," "if the father's brother's feelings have changed," standing as these persons.

This makes it possible for us to observe, not speculate. The constellation also makes it possible for us to get to know the client better. When he takes part in the constellation, we can observe his movements, we have his words and our own feelings from the field at our disposal. These elements enable deep insights into relevant mechanisms. The client, standing in the constellation, is often surprised by what he feels, because it goes beyond his memories and previous ideas.

Rose had problems in her relationships with men. Her father had died suddenly when she had been a teenager. She said she missed him very much. But standing in front of the father's representative, she could not accept him as a father. She did not look him in the face, she said she looked "between his legs." To the suggestion that she should say, "I accept you as a father," she replied, "But I want to make love with him." She said that she had washed her father's hair and back, that she had been happy to do it, even though she had felt uncomfortable. The client "missed her father." But what father? If I had just talked to her, maybe I would have accepted the fact that since she missed him, she recognized her father, loved him, and valued him. In other words, that she had no problem with her father. The constellation showed that she nursed a grievance against her father for leaving her, for dying. It also showed her sexual entanglement in this relationship. How much would I have had to talk to her to make such a controversial assumption?

Constellations provide an objectified view, because we have a wide range of complementary data at our disposal. The therapist has more than what the client tells him. He also has a broader picture of the relationship, and through representation he has access to the feelings of the people forming them. He can also access the client's emotions and attitude on an ongoing basis. For example, I stood in front of the client as a representative of her cousin, who sexually abused her in her childhood, and wondered what the solution was. I knew that a bond is established between a victim and a perpetrator, but in this case, this knowledge did not lead to a solution. I offered the client words of strength saying that she had been a child and that she left the guilt with the perpetrator. This, however, did not soothe her emotions.

I alternately tested internally what I felt as the cousin, what the client could feel, and what was happening between them. I also wondered how to link this all together to find a solution. Then I understood. I asked the client to say to her cousin, "We did it together." Although I had previously insisted on leaving the guilt with the cousin, now I noticed that the woman left "too much" of it, however strange it sounds. This sentence did bring change and relief. It is not that the perpetration was actually evenly distributed—the client remained a child and the perpetrator remained guilty—but it turned out to be important for the client to indicate her own part (she added, "Well, I didn't run away, although I could"). This was a discovery that I certainly would not have made during a simple conversation. It was only by sensing the cousin's attitude, confronting the client with him, listening to her in this situation, reading her emotions, and thinking what would ease the tension in this case, that I could figure out a solution.

During group constellations, we have representatives at our disposal, who in a way verify the therapist's concepts. The picture of the system emerges from the interaction of many minds, together with their sensitivity and ability for insight. The representatives form a group of interconnected elements, and the final picture results not from individual speculation but from a spontaneous combination of movements, feelings, and associations of many people. This, however, has nothing to do with a discussion or "brainstorming," there are no disputes or differences of opinion. At the end of the constellation, all the representatives find their place and form a coherent whole, one picture. The totality of the picture protects the therapist from making any fundamental mistakes in understanding the client's problem. For when we use a detached element in our thinking—for example, that the client's professional problems result from his childlike fear of the aggressive father—we can easily relate it to the person's life and get an apparent explanation. However, when we have at our disposal the multitude of feelings and behaviors of different family members, then we are not able to build a simple explanation offhand, to match all the elements. If, however, despite this, a coherent picture emerges, it is most likely correct.

Representation as a Source of Cognition

When we see how easily the representatives enter different psychophysical states, we can realize the power of systemic impact. How much greater is the impact it must have on the real member of the system. Being a representative has broadened my understanding of a child's mental states when his parents are in conflict, possible emotions in an incest situation, feelings of an adopted child, and feelings of a child during a cesarean section. I remember the state of erotic arousal and attraction while representing a man strongly attached to his mother. It gave me a picture of these, usually repressed, unconscious feelings. I would never have thought they are so unambiguous.

In another constellation, I represented a father who had a close, perhaps incestuous relationship with his daughter. In this constellation, both the mother and daughter had positive feelings for the father. As the father, I radiated love for them. In my real life, I have never felt anything like that. In the constellation, I was fully open both erotically and emotionally. I felt an incredible openness of the heart, from which deep affection for the daughter and, less so, for her mother flowed. This was the strongest feeling—in the psychophysical sense—of love I have ever experienced in my life. Here someone could say that I felt "something that was mine." But even if that was the case, the surprising intensity of that feeling should be explained. And that is not all. When we later shared our impressions, the representative of the daughter, described the same feelings and confessed that she had never felt such love in her life. She was a young girl, and I remember her abashment when she told me about it.

The constellation in which I represented a child of conflicted parents also made me think. It seemed like the situation was not dramatic yet, but as the child I felt I was falling into a black hole, complete emptiness and loneliness. Such an experience makes one realize that the internal state can be very different from what one sees. And it is this, above all, that influences the individual and shapes his destiny.

What else can I add? I represented one of the two *in vitro* fertilized egg cells. There were two, because one was expected to die, and I was that cell. There was an inner scream inside me because nobody saw me; I did not exist for the parents. What could this mean on an "ontic" level? At one of the training sessions someone asked if knowledge about the effects of abortion could help to solve the social conflict around this issue. Then one of the trainees said that after she had represented an aborted child and felt the unpleasant sensation of the body being stretched, the issue ceased to be a dilemma for her.

What actually are these sensations: is it real pain, real fear, panic? Can a representative experience the same as a man murdered in a gas chamber felt? In my opinion, these sensations consist of three components, in different proportions. First, there are specific physical sensations, for example, a feeling of suffocation, pain in some part of the body, and numbness. Second, emotions: sadness, fear, and loneliness. Third, there comes a certain understanding of a given situation, an awareness that what you are feeling is a sign of someone else's true sensations. When these three components come together in us, we can say that we know what the person felt and how difficult or terrible it was. Certainly, the physical sensations are incomparably weaker than they must have been in the real situation. Emotions are also not that strong, although sometimes their intensity surprises.

Interesting information (both from a psychological and historical point of view) about their sensations was shared by the participants of Hellinger's workshop in Russia. Stalin's representative said:

> When the constellation began, the strange thing was that I did not see any faces or eyes. I perceived them all as if they had had no heads. It made me feel like I had no human emotions. [. . .] This energy here was strange, it made me blind. It was like a stagnation, not a flow. [. . .] Under the influence of this force, I saw everyone not individually, separated from one another, but as a mass. They were not humans, but cells or even creatures without reason, something completely primitive.
>
> Very rarely did something human awaken in my soul. [. . .] Later, when I made contact with the people, and I saw their faces and eyes, I became a human again, I turned into a human again. [. . .]

> It was important for me to stand in the center first. Then it was important to throw other people in the center [this move symbolized Stalin's authority]. That was not a personal feeling. I often noticed that I was looking over people's heads, at the horizon. As if I was led by something that came from there. [. . .] I wasn't angry, I wasn't vicious. It was something else that I can't understand. Then I understood that I needed someone in the service, someone who could do the task, collect and throw people in.
>
> He tried to escape, which made me laugh, because I kept an eye on what was happening outside the circle. [. . .] I had an impression that it was Trotsky, murdered in Mexico. I had this strange feeling: "What do you mean? Who are you trying to do that with? Who are you trying to do battle with?" When suddenly someone came up to me from behind, I had a warm feeling. I wanted to get this thing out of my back. I didn't want it to affect me. [. . .] Before throwing people from the outer circle to the inner one, I felt that my heart would break. I thought my heart would burst and I would have a heart attack. It was an impression that this energy had closed everything else for me. (Hellinger 2014, 58–59)[3]

What do these feelings and thoughts tell us about Stalin? About paranoia or psychopathy? About history? One might think that they are only projections of the representative's associations and historical knowledge. However, based on other cases, we know that constellations show deep inner states of people and their systemic conditioning.

Insights and Visions

The insights formulated by the therapist in constellations concern, for instance, the basic orders in the family, relationships between the attitude of its members and their life, and relationships between diseases and systemic dynamics. For example, Hellinger's sentence: "No one can be healthy without a bond with their mother" is an insight. When such conclusions, that are in line with the orders of love, are expressed, there is a particular sense of adequacy, we are positive that what we say is right and universal. Bertold Ulsamer wrote that it was a surprising experience for him to facilitate constellations, because in some situations and moments:

> [. . .] authority grew in me out of somewhere. I was so unexpectedly sure of what I perceived at that moment that I could take the risk of representing it to the outside with all power. This was new to me and had never happened before in this form. The more familiar I became with the work, the more obvious it became for me that this certainty would appear again and again in me. [. . .] Therefore,

my guess is that it is the power of the "knowing field" that creates or supports the phenomenon of authority. (Ulsamer 1999, 129–30)[4]

That authority is built from insights that Bert Hellinger refers to so often. To some extent, they are available to everyone. When I talk about the issues arising from the orders of love, the listeners and I feel that they are indisputable. An insight concerns a particular matter and can be limited to one or a few sentences. When I continue the topic for too long, after a while I realize that these are no longer insights but deliberations. I feel it physically; there is a kind of slight confusion in my head. This happened, for example, when I let myself extrapolate the systemic orders too far to politics, or when I wanted to consider gender differences in too much detail.

The therapist experiences insights also in a narrower sense. These do not concern general truths, but the situation of the client. We can call it reading the client's field. There is nothing mystical about it. Some problems or attitudes can be felt already during the conversation. This is the knowledge that goes beyond what the client says, even beyond what he says between the lines. Insights can take the form of some kind of association, a sentence heard in the head, and a feeling that we then interpret, or a vision.

In my work with Theresa, whose problem was her fears, I represented someone from the past. As this person I turned to the wall, to the more distant past, and "saw" that "there were many people there." I wanted to reach out to them, and I had a vision that they were doing it too, they were grabbing my hands. I told the client about it, and it turned out that she "saw" it too. This image brought her peace, but only partial. I wondered what else could matter here. First of all, I had to understand what was happening to the client. How? By empathizing with her state while confronting with what came to me from the family. And I understood. These people, it was "too much" for her, their "presence" caused fear, which made it impossible for her to take strength from the ancestors (obviously the whole process did not happen just now, but already in her childhood).

So I said to "them" that they only partly belonged to her family system and had their own systems, that now they turned to them and went their separate ways (I need to mention that I did not treat this as "escorting the souls" but as a work with the client's system and internal images). The client who bowed before this past, said it was "a beautiful sight to see them go to their systems." It was clear to me that she "saw" the same thing as me.

What does it mean to "see" in such cases? I refer to this form of perception as semi-images, or something on the border between visualizations and feelings, which I would describe as kinesthetic. It is like feeling somebody, who is standing next to us. Leaving aside visual, auditory, or thermal sensations,

I think most people would agree that there is some bodily "feeling of presence." So there is nothing unusual about these semi-images in the visual layer. There is only a spontaneous, but persistent image.

Hellinger sometimes said, "The insights that came to me," "The insights that were given to me," which might suggest he was some kind of prophet. The greatness of the method he developed, however, is that insights can also be available to other therapists and to some extent to anyone who takes part in a constellation. Selecting the sentence of strength that is right for the given person, in the right moment, is also a kind of insight. That is what Hellinger says about it:

> When you really open yourself to a situation and wait, then a decisive sentence comes to you. When you say it, you do not have to do anything else. It has a very special power and works through itself.
>
> Some time ago, I was visited by a man who climbs with delinquent adolescents and facilitates family constellations. We talked to each other and I told him, "Wait a minute, I want to find a sentence for you to say to the teenagers when climbing." And the sentence was, "It ends here." This is a multi-layered sentence because it leaves the question of what ends and where it ends open. For example, it could concern the behaviors that led them to prison. In Rome, I said to a woman, "Someone who wants to live according to their wishes, misses out on life."
>
> [. . .] I focus on the person and on their system and I wait until a sentence comes that changes everything for everyone. You cannot think of such a sentence and you cannot search for it. You just wait, you are open and suddenly it is there, quite surprisingly. When we follow the soul like this, we have also another experience. We reach the depths of the soul, where we meet some dragons. At first we think they are ugly and evil. But they guard a special treasure. If we face them and reconcile with them, they lead us to something essential. (Hellinger and Walper, n.d.)[5]

MISTAKES IN UNDERSTANDING AND FACILITATING CONSTELLATIONS

Innovation and Eclecticism

The method of family constellations—provided that the therapist adheres to the systemic orders—offers many variants and styles of work that can be equally helpful to clients. I am far from criticizing other therapists, but I would like to point out a few ways of applying and understanding constellations which, even if they are not completely incorrect, do not enable to achieve full therapeutic effects. Sometimes they do not support the image of constellations. To better systematize these mistakes, I have given them names.

There are therapists who try hard to implement their own innovations in constellations. However, these do not stem from the fact that they have discovered something really new. Ulsamer argues that simplicity is problematic for some therapists, so they need some "garnish," while others want to bring into constellations what they were previously associated with, such as Gestalt therapy or psychodrama (Ulsamer 2001, 133–35). Other therapists are pressed by their egos, and they need to add something new so that systemic constellations are not so "Hellingerian" and look like their own method.

Some therapists find it difficult to understand the completeness of constellations as a method. They want to see them as one of the techniques that can at most be an introduction or basis for further therapy. They think that there is something inappropriate about the fact that, as one of them wrote, "we come to a group session, have constellations and finish." The same author also maintained that Hellinger's constellations "are a therapeutic technique (like any other) that can be used in a wider treatment process, then they are absolutely justifiable" (Zdrada 2017, 217).[6] In fact, constellations are not just a therapeutic technique. They bring about the orders of love, and this makes important pathogenic factors immediately disappear, enabling many clients to say goodbye to the problem forever. Therefore, a constellation session is a closed whole that does not need any external support.

Of course, in some cases, constellations can be combined with regular long-term therapy, but for most clients this is not necessary. Another thing is that a constellation does not have to be one, and one can meet the client many times (which usually takes place at intervals of several months and sometimes several years).

However, some feel the obligation or need to combine constellations with other methods, claiming that only then are they really effective and safe. One of the therapists combines constellations with the Hawaiian practice of Ho'oponopono because she believes that this helps her avoid the negative aspects of the generally positive process of constellations. These negative aspects are, in her opinion, "leaving" the participants with difficult or traumatic information obtained during the constellation. The therapist cites the following example:

> A child of one and a half years old died in unexplained circumstances in a family. No one could explain the event, but the energy of the child's death had a negative impact on all members of the family. Thanks to constellations we were able to find out the cause of his death. It turned out that the client's grandfather

> inadvertently dropped the child he cared for on the floor, contributing to his death. Although the energy of this tragedy, on the family level, was purified, the granddaughter could not cope with the thought that her grandfather was an unintentional killer. (in: Osiński 2017, 69)[7]

According to the therapist's account, this awareness was traumatizing for the client, and the therapist had to deal with this "trauma" using a different method. She claims that during therapy, the "process of purification" can only be initiated in prepared and aware people, the unprepared, taking part in a constellation for the first time, may not be able to cope with some information.

There is a certain truth in this statement. I do not think that Hellinger's work could cause traumas to clients, but it is true that in the later period of his work, he did not focus on what I describe as working with the inner attitude, that is, on what happens in the client's mind. It seems that this is the aspect that the therapist wants to deal with more using Ho'oponopono. But it can also be dealt with using constellations. In the example above, in order to complete the process, the client should have taken into the heart both the deceased child and the grandfather, for which constellations provide excellent tools.

Prophesying

Ann was in a relationship with a man who showed no desire to deepen the relationship. She broke up with him many times, and then started the relationship again. Some time ago she met another man, but the relationship with him did not quite suit her. She said she needed to definitively end the first relationship and wanted to find a new partner. The therapist wrote the names of both men on two sheets of paper, the third sheet represented a potential new man. She put the sheets on the floor with the blank side upwards so that Ann could not see where each sheet was. She then instructed the client to stand on each sheet and describe her feelings. Finally, she turned the sheets over. It turned out that when she was standing on the piece of paper marked with the name of the man with whom she had had the longest relationship, she described the feelings of a strong attraction to that piece of paper. In the other cases, her feelings were much weaker. The therapist interpreted it in the following way: Ann should stay with that man, fight for their relationship, she also said about the man's "true love." After some time, Ann called me for an appointment, as the issue was not solved at all.

Constellations make it possible for us to test relationships and draw conclusions about them, but this requires great caution in formulating judgments and refraining from suggesting what decisions our clients should make. The only thing that the described constellation brought is the confirmation of the fact that the client was attached to that man. The idea that the client should stand on the pieces of paper representing the men was a technical mistake. Was she supposed to represent them in this way or to examine her attitude toward them? Or both? By working in this way, we blur the picture, and we do not get to the point. The client did not get any new information and did not realize anything.

We must not change a constellation into a mantic technique or clairvoyance. As Daan van Kampenhout writes, the soul does not store any "stories or anecdotes," but rather "traces and structures derived from experience" (Kampenhout 2006, 214).[8] He cites an example of the client who, through a constellation, wants to make sure that he was molested as a child. In such a constellation, the representatives will not be completely free, because "whatever they feel or experience will determine the answer to be 'Yes' or 'No,' and this is a big responsibility," while carrying out the constellation "when all participants know that a specific question about the incestuous family history has been asked, will turn the constellation into a projection screen" (Kampenhout 2006, 214–15).[9] The wish for the constellation to answer a specific question would block the openness to what is revealed, which is necessary in this method. The client should expect changes and improvement of his health, not satisfaction of his curiosity.

Mixing Up of Roles

One therapist worked with a client in such a way that she made her stand as her own mother so that she could "see what kind of relationship the mother had with her father." Of course, this session did not have any positive effects. The therapist's intervention was a simple way to get the client involved in the matters that did not concern her and to cause her to violate the hierarchy. The client should rather not represent any of his family members. It is best if the client remains himself in the constellation, and the other persons are represented by the therapist or representatives.

In the example above, the procedure suggested by the therapist may have resulted from some kind of transference and the therapist may have realized the client's Oedipal fantasies or her own. What could the client learn from this? What could she work through? It was a rather straight path to get even more confused.

Excess of Abstraction

In some constellations, nonpersonal and abstract elements are represented, such as "illnesses," "death," "life," "birth," "fate," as well as elements such as "anger" or the "inner child," that represent the suppressed aspects of the client's self. The representatives of these elements have the same task as when they represent people, so they communicate their feelings and move. However, while "fate" or the "inner child" are directly related to Hellinger's method, bringing in representatives of "chakras" or the "Higher Ego" goes far from the foundations of the method, if it is not meaningless at all.

This does not mean that the use of any abstract and nonpersonal elements in a constellation makes no sense. On the contrary, they are sometimes necessary. However, one should remember what Hellinger himself argues—that behind these elements, there are usually people from the system (Ulsamer 1999, 154, Ulsamer 2001, 245). The constellation should first of all direct toward relationships with real people (including the deceased ones and unborn children), and abstract elements should be used in moderation and without unnecessary hypostatizing. A constellation in which the client's "inner child," "soul," "anger," "future," and "love" will be placed at the same time next to the client's representative will definitely not be an effective one. Could anyone understand any of this?

Daimonization

I use the term "daimonization" to describe the tendency to see supernatural beings in place of human beings. Although this does not apply to constellations, a good example of this tendency is given by Jungian psychoanalyst Clarissa Pinkola Estés, who claims that when she was four years old, she met the archetypal Great Mother at the lake:

> And that's when I first saw her, the lady in the water coming toward me. [. . .] I cannot explain this: I felt I was seeing a long-lost relative that I so loved, and had missed so dearly for an eternity. I was so glad to see her I tried to run farther into the water toward her, but she was calling to me, "No, no! Don't run toward me. I came to run after you. Turn around, run away from me! She was playing a game with me. I understood now, and turned before the next wave crashed. I ran laughing, heavy booted and all, falling palms down through water that had no bottom, water going straight up my nose, but I rose choking, coughing, slog-running some more. (Estés 2013, 10–11)

For the constellation therapist, such words are a signal that in fact, it could have been some dead relative who appeared in a spontaneous visualization. The child risked by following this person, but she—as is usually the case in constellations—did not expect this movement, and turned the girl back. After this incident, Estés was rebuked by her family, which she later assessed as a misunderstanding of her experience.

Estés would probably consider the above conclusions to be a reduction of the peak experience resulting from the need to "pare down the numinous, the infinitely larger, the unfamiliar, the unknown, the 'other,' the different" (Estés 2013, 18). But is it not equally common to "magnify" our experiences and add a supernatural touch to them? Some people want to see unearthly beings where there actually are relationships with humans. In constellations, we should not go to such areas, because experience shows that we achieve the greatest effects by keeping feet on the ground and referring to relationships with humans and not with angels.

Equating

During constellations, we should avoid equating two different persons. This kind of error can occur when we are too concerned about the theory of reincarnation. The therapist may claim that a person "has the same soul" as his great-grandfather or some unidentified figure appearing in the constellation. Instead of trying to resolve the entanglement, he will reinforce it, suggesting that two people are one and the same. Where there is identification (entanglement) with someone from the past, this constellation facilitator will see the migration of the soul.

Without considering whether reincarnation exists or not, I would like to point to the dangers of being overly attached to this concept. Therapist Jasmin Schober-Howorka, who combines systemic constellations and the idea of reincarnation, maintains that her method extends "beyond our ancestors" and discovers "the causal correlations from earlier times" (Schober-Howorka 2012, 27). She argues that through the prism of reincarnation one can understand things that previously seemed accidental, for instance, why something burdens a given person and not his sister or brother. She explains that rejecting parents may result from our bad experiences with them in previous incarnations. She also hypothesizes that we choose our own fate, so even difficult situations are our choice, and not the accidental activity of the environment. This approach can be a way to take responsibility for one's life more fully. However, there are also dangers hidden in it. This understanding may lead to the client's confusion as to the extent of his responsibility and cause difficulties in acknowledging the system hierarchy. Besides, explanations of this kind are not reflected in the client's directly observable reality.

Transgenerational Sins

What is transmitted in the family and affects the next generations? It may be that everything is written in the Akashic records, but the practice of constellations shows that only some events and attitudes are really important for the next generations.[10] Some authors tend to see transgenerational factors too broadly, as the sum of all "violations" on the part of our ancestors. As one of them writes, trying to refer to the principles of Hellinger's therapy:

> We grow and develop—in the literal sense—in the vast field of the multigenerational family. According to this, for example, what happened in my great-grandmother's marriage—whether she was a happy wife and mother or suffered—has a definite meaning for my mental and physical health as her great-grandson. Similarly, depending on whether my grandfather was an alcoholic, troublemaker and womanizer, or a well-balanced man, full of humor and optimism, my life as his grandson may be shaped. (Karpowicz 2007, 62)[11]

Perhaps the fact that the "grandfather was a womanizer" has some effect on the grandson, but this question is not within the scope of systemic constellations, just as the fact whether he was "full of humor and optimism." This is not how we look at transgenerational factors. We see them above all as a violation of the orders of love (exclusion of someone, failure to accept a parent, parentification, negation of a bond, and rejection of perpetrators or victims), as a transmission of traumas impossible to assimilate mentally (war, murder, genocide, and death of a child), as a legacy of someone's great guilt. It is primarily these factors that are transmitted in the family, and that we work with during constellations. Of course, such events can cause that the grandfather is full of sadness or anger, but this is not what we focus on in this method. The beginning of the problem was not his "unpleasant" personality traits, but certain events and systemic dynamics.

Exorcizing

This mistake consists in perceiving some of our ancestors as "ghosts" that can "cling to us." Some people say, taking this seriously, that the "dead object" to something, that the "grandmother has tagged along with" someone, or that something "bad from the dead has been passed on to you." This view is followed by attempts to "detach" or even "chase" the dead away. Schober-Howorka claims that one can not only be identified with the ancestor, but also "possessed" by him (Schober-Howorka 2012). In my work, I have never observed such a phenomenon.

What model is closer to the truth? It is the soul of the child (client) that "clings" to the deceased—it gravitates toward them and toward the past associated with them. Every "casting out" of the soul of the deceased goes against the orders of love, which consists in accepting and reintegrating the members into the family system. Seeing someone as demonic and deserving to be removed has nothing to do with the principle of systemic constellations, according to which the equality and unity of all people is fundamental.

At the workshop, which was attended by one of my clients, the facilitators did not solve his problems because they considered that his ancestors "opposed" his professional decisions. The dynamics that the client and I found out were not far from what he had learned at that workshop, but I focused on the client's attitude and his attitude to his ancestors. In constellations, there is no such thing as ancestors who oppose, who have their own opinion that should be respected. Ancestors do not mind our choices. If in some way they "oppose" something, it is just breaking the family's orders of love. When these are respected, ancestors become silent.

Occultism

Some facilitators use introductory ceremonies, "energy-clearing" rituals after the session, amulets, and requests addressed to ancestors (Carnabucci and Anderson 2012, 172). There is no rationale behind this. We need neither to induce the family field in any special way, nor to "protect ourselves" from the influence of the "spirits of the dead," nor in some special way to release representatives from their roles or to "cleanse" the room. Implementing "protective" rituals for representatives makes constellations strange, adding little or nothing to them. It can also be a veil for mistakes made or for unfinished constellation processes. The vast majority, if not every properly facilitated constellation, ends up with a kind of energy drop, "scattering" of the field, and a feeling of "being released" in representatives. To facilitate the completion of the process, all you have to do is touch the representative and clearly say that this is the end of the constellation. Prayers, rituals, or altars for ancestors make constellations back to nonempirical religious practices and the traditional image of the spirits of the dead, which does not correspond to what we see in systemic constellations. And suggesting that some special protective practices should be used may make potential clients fear.

At this point, I should also mention the tendency of some people to see good or bad energy everywhere. The "energy" unknown to science undoubtedly exists. However, it seems that systemic constellations have brought about a lot of order and understanding here, showing that the most important are the energies of our family. If we put them in order, other energies turn out to be less important. Some, however, cannot do without, generally idle, pondering of the multiplicity of energetic influences and confusing the essential with the vestigial.

During a workshop I attended, one of the participants asked, "Does the person because of whom I almost died twice belong to the system?" she probably referred to the fact that killers belong to the system. In a very confusing way, she explained what she meant, saying something about suffocation. Eventually, it turned out that when she met one man, she choked twice in a row. Gerhard Walper, who ran that workshop, told her, "These are delusions." I cite this example to underline that—although they address energy influences—systemic constellations do not mingle everything with everything. A person we meet is unlikely to suck energy out of us or cast a spell. And if this happens, it is probably because we have triggered some aspects of our own systemic situation that had already been present before.

According to Hellinger, some diseases result from a "curse," especially atopic dermatitis in children. However, if we take a closer look at what situations he had in mind, we can see that "curses" work because they are caused by people who belong to the system—parent's ex-partners, those who nurse anger or grudge. An illness is an unconscious and psychophysical reaction of children who internally follow the person who "cursed" them. "Casting a curse" by the former partner and his children is simply their bad thinking about the future. And experiencing the curse can be understood as a result of the unconscious relationship between the child and the person who suffered the loss.

Redundant Comments

This mistake usually results from hubris. The therapist wants to mark his existence more than is advisable and sufficient. During one constellation, the client was a woman whose father died in strange circumstances. She was convinced it was a murder. When I represented her father, I wanted to say at some point that it did not look like a homicide to me. But I refrained. First of all, I was not at all sure what the dynamics related to the father showed me, and second, I asked myself, "What will this give her?" Would I say this for her good, or just to demonstrate my abilities?

Bert Hellinger recommends asking oneself similar questions. If the therapist speaks too much, it is possible that he will go beyond what is real, toward his own fantasies and unconscious needs. Therefore, he should weigh his words and use them very moderately. Especially those who carry many unconscious conflicts pose a threat to the therapeutic process, when they start talking. That is why they should remain silent, then they can facilitate constellations well and help their clients.

Some of the therapists' words are not needed by anyone but themselves. These are words that go beyond the orders of love, and the therapist is credible only if he adheres to the orders. Sometimes, the facilitator's statements are built on aggression and disrespect for the client. One of the therapists said to her client, "How many more people do you want to die in your family?" There were indeed several deaths in the client's family, possibly systemically related. However, the client herself was not the manager of that system. Whatever her inner attitude might have been—perhaps annoying to someone—such questions do not help to solve the problem. The therapist is not the client's educator or judge. If he has an irresistible inclination toward these functions, he should change his profession.

ANSWER TO OBJECTIONS

Systemic constellations, which are developing and gaining more and more clients, have not escaped the attention of therapists from other schools. Among them there are those who are aware of the fundamental importance of family entanglements and suggest that their patients go to systemic constellations, and there are those who do not want to agree with the principles of this method. Are their objections, sometimes formulated as concerns about patients who undergo new and "scientifically unproven" therapy, justified?

Some psychotherapeutic methods are presented as scientific, other as non-scientific. However, no significant therapeutic method has been developed as a result of systematic scientific research. Therapeutic systems such as psychoanalysis, Gestalt therapy (by no means based on Gestalt psychology; Henle 1986, 22 et seq.), transactional analysis, family therapy, and many other, are not based on any strictly scientific theory. If any theories of academic science are compatible with or support these methods, they are created later and do not cover the entirety of the issues. Behavior therapy based on the conclusions of researchers like Ivan Pavlov and Burrhus Frederic Skinner could be considered an exception. Their research on animal behavior had all the attributes of a scientific method. However, extrapolation of these results to humans, and their subsequent implementation into the process of therapy, entailed enormous simplifications (e.g., Breland and Breland 1961).

Therapists' objections are mostly due to their attachment to their own method. They are unable to see that procedures completely different from those they know can also produce therapeutic effects. When systemic constellations were presented at one congress "several psychodrama practitioners left the room in disgust because they were convinced that the process they were watching was ineffective, wrong and invalid" (Carnabucci and Anderson 2012, 11). Of course, they did not let themselves see how things really are.

Many therapists equate the laborious and long-lasting contact with the client with ethics and giving him a sense of security. It is difficult for them to accept that a one-time meeting can be at least as supportive, honest, and healing as years of psychotherapy. This state of affairs breaks the paradigm built up over decades that "real therapy" is long and difficult, and that the client is more or less helpless in the course of it, needing the therapist's watchful eye.

All codes of ethics for psychotherapists have been developed based on this understanding of the therapeutic process. Because the patient was involved in long-lasting contact with the therapist, this raised many concerns as to whether some kind of abuse would occur. The more so as the therapeutic contact concerns the most intimate matters and usually takes place without witnesses. Additionally, psychoanalysis proved that the relationship between two people is a very unclear situation in which unconscious drives and fantasies are involved, both on the part of the patient and the therapist.

The guidelines of the psychotherapist's code of ethics—which refers to the "psychotherapy process"—are addressed by one of the therapists who criticizes systemic constellations:

> The Hellinger's procedure, based on a one-time contact with a person experiencing a family constellation, does not fulfil the criterion of a "psychotherapeutic process." If the described family constellations are not based on a process then they make it practically impossible to examine this method as psychotherapy, and what follows, to examine it also in the context of the code of ethics. It is also difficult to talk about "ethical responsibility of a psychotherapist toward participants of the therapeutic process" if there is no process. (Talarczyk 2011, 71)

The author's line of reasoning is that since there is just one therapeutic meeting, there is no "process" and therefore constellations cannot be considered psychotherapy, which in turn means that the ethical dimension cannot be used to evaluate the constellation therapists' conduct. As one can see, the whole problem starts with the fact that the meeting is only one. The author does not mention mental processes, therapeutic effects, necessary training, self-experience, theory of formation of disorders, sensitivity toward the client, and other elements that cause that we can refer to constellations as psychotherapy. Since a constellation is a one-time event, it does not fit into the familiar paradigm. And instead of reflecting on the limitations of this paradigm, she tries to discredit the method.

In 2004, the so-called "Potsdam Declaration on Systemic Constellation Work" was initiated by Arist von Schlippe, chairman of the German Systemic Society (*Systemische Gesellschaft*), and published (Hellinger and Heilmann 2018, 249 et seq.). Prior to that, Schlippe wrote an open letter to Bert Hellinger, in which he both emphasized the strengths of constellation work and pointed out that Hellinger used "simplified ideas," "generalized" the issues concerning men and women, and believed that he had gained special knowledge. All this allegedly undermined systemic therapy, in which Schlippe included systemic constellations.[12] I will address the statement itself, abstracting from the personal and professional motives of its author—a person whose career is closely connected with traditional systemic therapy.

Schlippe formulates the following objections against constellations: neglecting the detailed reason for visiting the therapist; neglecting work strictly focused on the client's problem; using mystifying phrases such as "something greater," "taken into service;" using overly generalized or dogmatic phrases such as "always when," "the only way"[13]; using potentially humiliating interventions and rituals of subordination; relationship between therapeutic intervention and a specific world view (regarding gender, parenthood, dual nationality issues); imagining that one person has better access to the truth than the other, which entails the lack of partnership based on cooperation.

Addressing this critique, I will refer not only to the work of Hellinger himself, but also to my own therapeutic practice. My style of work is very different from that of Hellinger, but I follow his findings strictly, that is why in refuting the critique of constellations I can refer to my own work. By the way, many of the misunderstandings about systemic constellations stem from equating Hellinger's style of work with the essence of the method.

Let us start with the alleged negligence of the client's reason for contacting the therapist. Indeed, in constellations, it is possible to work without any initial interview with the client. When working individually, I can ask the client to stand up and—to make it easier for myself to enter the role—I can take a piece of paper and put it on the floor and say: "This piece of paper represents what you're coming with/what's important here/the problem." Then I can stand on this piece of paper and follow my movement. In fact, I could start any constellation this way, which does not mean that this single represented position would be enough for us. Usually, I would bring in the client's parents and other people. But it could be that the client would immediately identify what or whom it is about, and such direct confrontation would prove to heal.

And what about the fact that in constellations we do not necessarily focus on the problem, or the expectations regarding the solution that the client has? This is because we are aware that the solution may lie in completely unexpected areas. The client comes to us because he, say, wants to be rich, and we offer him to work on the relationship with his mother or to take his deceased brother into his heart. Not addressing the issue of money at all. Do we not pay attention to his expectations? I personally apply the technical rule that at the end of the constellation I return to the client's original question or expectation if we did not work on it directly. In a case like the above, I add "money." I stand in its place and the client stands opposite. Then we see how the dynamics has changed.

The objections regarding generalizations, the vision of parenthood, the understanding of femininity and masculinity, dual nationality, and the like result from adhering to the constructivist approach of systemic therapy. In this therapy, it has been assumed as standard that there are "many individual truths," "everyone has their own interpretation of the world," and conclusions should be reached in dialogue with the client. These principles are justifiable and the therapy based on them makes sense. In constellations, however, we have discovered a seemingly contradictory, though probably complementary, level of our human existence. There are things beyond interpretation, things that affect us, whether we want it or not. If someone was adopted, then even though he is fully convinced that his only and true parents are his caregivers, this fact will affect him. Even if he totally believes that it does not matter who begat him, but who raised him, it will not change anything. Something deep inside him will demand that he acknowledge the importance of his real parents, and if he does not do so, the problem will be taken over by his children. In classic systemic therapy, we would have to take these views and feelings of the client seriously, and we would have no right to interfere. Unless, at some point, he would tell us that they are becoming a source of suffering for him. This is different in constellations, during which we can reach deeper causal relationships and the client's hidden feelings. Such a person would usually find out and feel quite easily that the biological parents do matter and that rejecting them affects his life.

Do we practice humiliating interventions in systemic constellations? I have never seen anything like this at any workshop, and none of my clients has ever said (or written on the Internet) that they felt humiliated. So what does the author of the declaration mean? Probably such elements of constellations as bowing or lying in front of one's parents. It is hard to figure out if there is anything else. Perhaps the situation when the representative of the perpetrator faces the client who was sexually abused? Consider lying in front of the parents in order to restore the hierarchy. Some clients find it difficult to acknowledge that their parents are parents and that they are "only" children. Interestingly, even if they want to do so, they feel that they are blocked by the images they remember when they had to be "big," support their depressed mother or take care of their drunken father. Then I often tell them: "I'll help you. Lie down on your stomach in front of your mother (representative), stretch your arms forward." Then I say, "Leave all the stories, feel like a child, your mother's child. Feel what comes from her, what comes from the mother to the child. Open up to it. You are small. She is big." And this exercise almost always helps. The hierarchy becomes rebuilt, which is experienced by the client as good and strengthening. This mechanism works regardless of his previous thinking.

It would be much easier to find "humiliations" in other forms of therapy. Eva Røine, a psychodrama therapist, describes a psychodrama of Inger, a woman who was raped by her father in childhood:

> With the utmost care, the director gradually guides the scene into the offensive act by relating how it was done. The therapist spreads the girl's legs while assuring her that she is not the father. [. . .]. The protagonist is then encouraged to fight against the father and told that this time it will work. After numerous

> seizures of vomiting, Inger started fighting her father. Soon she was screaming and shouting words that she had been carrying inside her throughout her life. (Røine 1997, 181)

I have no grounds to disbelieve that such interventions produce a therapeutic effect. However, in constellations, our proceedings are incomparably more cautious and not so invasive. There is no reason to spread someone's thighs and imitate the act of rape. We base our conduct on mutual relations and feelings, and not on actions designed to remind of old traumas.

The frequent objection is pointing to the alleged authoritarianism present in Hellinger's assertions. This results from looking at his work in a superficial way. Take as an example Hellinger's work with a therapist treating a refugee from Ethiopia. This man fought against government troops in his country, and the therapist, being under the influence of transference, sympathized with him. Hellinger said that his soul was with the people he had killed. During the constellation, the man's representative lay down by the representatives of the victims. Hellinger said that this was the only solution, that this was "the only way he could regain his dignity" and that it would be even better if "he went back to his country and was shot." When the therapist objected, Hellinger replied, "I mean the images and whether or not you can see yourself in them. Not what he will actually do or what he can do" (Hellinger 2008b, 230).[14] The same applies when Hellinger tells someone that he should undo the adoption or not start a family. Against all appearances—and even Hellinger's assertions that he really means it—these are not absolute recommendations. They are images that clearly show things as they are. There is a paradox here—the more the client is able to agree to them internally, the greater the area of freedom opens up to him, and then he can do something else.

Interestingly, in conventional family therapy, therapeutic gurus have long been talked about. Salvador Minuchin said that it is practiced by people "who do not shy away from the pleasure of playing to audiences and being charismatic. This is a field with a lot of very narcissistic people who enjoy that game" (Simon 1992, 79). Well-known therapists displayed personality traits and style of work that went far beyond Hellinger's alleged authoritarianism or manipulations. Minuchin himself distorted the truth to disrupt the balance in a marriage for therapeutic purposes. He commented on his interventions, saying that if someone "versed in ethics" criticized him for being unfair, they would be right (Simon 1992, 80). Carl Whitaker teased people to experience the "craziness" and "challenged all the rules and conventions of therapy. At various stages of his career, he has bottle-fed his patients, arm-wrestled with them, refused to allow them to talk, even fallen asleep on them" (Simon 1992, 99–100). He also believed that "the therapist's job is to stir up things in the family without having an equal responsibility for resolving them" (Simon 1992, 103). I do not judge these therapists in the slightest, I had no contact with their clients, and they would be the only ones to express binding opinions. However, I would not want to use a method that gives such freedom in choosing techniques.

Franz Ruppert uses the knowing field, representing the traumatized parts of the patient. However, he does not recognize the orders of love. He writes:

> Therapies can even help a client's survival strategies [pathological strategies] if they convey illusory experiences of attachment, contact and love from the parents, which in reality did not happen, and which could not happen because the parents are incapable of constructive attachment and love because of their own traumatization. [. . .] Another widespread survival strategy is to imagine the removal of the experience of lack of love by internally bonding with those who are deceased, for example, grandparents who died prematurely, or a sibling. [. . .] It is also a popular survival strategy to reduce traumatizing experiences of violence and perpetrator-victim dynamics to a simple experience of loss, which makes reconciliation possible with relatives who are actually the perpetrators. (Ruppert et al. 2016, 48–50)

Ruppert reduces the orders of love to an ideology and illusion on the part of therapists and irrational ways of dealing with trauma on the part of clients. However, these orders are a fact and manifest themselves without any knowledge on the part of the client or suggestions made by the therapist; most clearly during silent family constellations. It is the representatives who reveal the need for reconciliation, not only between parents and children, but even between murderers and their victims. Apparently Ruppert understands love in a colloquial way, which is why he concludes that since it "wasn't there," it will never happen. However, in constellations, we discover another love, hidden under the surface of our daily family relationships. This love is actually a kind of life energy—it flows from the ancestors no matter how much they have closed themselves off as a result of their own traumas. And to this love we can always open ourselves. It is also what turns out to be most important.

Also the fact that one can be "in the care" of the departed is not a survival strategy. It is the experience of thousands of people, which we do not lead to by any persuasion or suggestion. It is created already when we imagine our ancestors behind our backs (of course, if we resolve the cause of our entanglement and blockade beforehand). It is a strong, energetic experience that has nothing to do with wishful thinking. It has also been known to members of traditional cultures for thousands of years.

Ruppert says:

> Some regard the abstract concept of parenthood as being much more important than actual parenthood, arguing that the person's own life came from his

> or her parents and they would not have been there at all otherwise. They are thereby drawing from a biological fact—it is true that without their parents these children would not have existed—a psychological conclusion: the parents do earn *per se* respect and appreciation, whatever they did to their children. "Respecting" parents then becomes a "law of nature." [. . .] But psychological givens do not result from biological facts. (Ruppert et al. 2016, 50)

This fact is not abstract. What is more, this kind of gratitude for life appears—albeit to a lesser extent—also toward parents' former partners who "made room" for children from the new relationship. On some level, they owe their lives to them. The requirement of respect for parents is indeed a kind of natural law. Contrary to what Ruppert says, our psyche is marked by the fact that it is these people who are the beginning of our lives. That life came to us through our parents is more than just a biological fact. It is an existential fact. The merit of systemic constellations is that they have shown that it has great psychological consequences.

NOTES

1. Bert Hellinger sometimes talked about the dead "who cling to us and drag us to death" (Hellinger and Nehrebecki 2012, 352; quotation translated from Polish). I think, however, that these statements are closer to a metaphor than a description of a real process. This is how one can experience one's particular bond with the deceased, but the main part of activity comes from the living. Besides, Hellinger referred primarily to the ones who died from a sudden death, who "do not know that they have passed away." Perhaps in such cases, there is some specific influence, but I have not observed it.
2. Also in the brain, social information is organized in a "cartographic" form, similar to mental maps of the environment. The information includes the distance between individuals, their status, affiliation, and so forth. It turns out that the same brain modules can control spatial navigation, time orientation, reasoning, memory, and social interactions (Shafer and Schiller 2020, 30 et seq.).
3. Quotation translated from Polish.
4. Quotation translated from German.
5. Quotation translated from German.
6. Quotation translated from Polish.
7. Quotation translated from Polish.
8. Quotation translated from Polish.
9. Quotation translated from Polish.
10. Akasha is one of the five elements in Hindu philosophy, a kind of ether. The Akashic Chronicle is a Hindu and esoteric concept saying that all events, information, all knowledge about man are recorded and potentially available.
11. Quotation translated from Polish.

12. He also cited press reports that described Hellinger as an extreme right-winger, even a Nazi (such issues as Hellinger's reflections on Adolf Hitler, "right-wing" views on the existence of differences between men and women, statements about Jews having nothing to do with antisemitism, and accidental living for some time in a building that had housed one of Hitler's many offices were mixed up here). This is all the more unfair as Hellinger kept away from Nazism during World War II, for which he was declared a "potential public enemy," literally: "potential folk pest" (German: *potenzieller Volksschädling*), which could have resulted in a death sentence for him (Hellinger and Heilmann 2018, 45).

13. Schlippe also points to Hellinger's allegedly spoken sentences like "punished with death" and "bad effect." Schlippe seems to suggest that in his work, Hellinger was driven by the judgments of his own conscience. This would obviously be non-therapeutic, and Hellinger never did so. Schlippe also refers to the phrase "forfeiting one's right" as raising his objections. In the early period of his work, Hellinger used to say that, for example, murderers in the family or mothers who gave their children away "forfeited their rights" (in the family system, toward children). Later, however, as he observed the movements of the spirit, which are directed toward everyone equally, he stopped using such expressions.

14. Quotations translated from Polish.is

Chapter 3

Therapeutic Effects of Constellations

THERAPEUTIC FACTORS

Systemic constellations are a process that has a great impact on the human psyche. Trying to break this whole process down into components, we can say that constellations work on two basic levels: first, they influence the client's mind, and second—the entire system. In other words, the constellation affects the client's consciousness, unconsciousness, and extraconsciousness, as I define the field of the family system. Consciousness and unconsciousness is the personal level, the narrowly understood "mind," while extraconsciousness is the systemic level.

When analyzing the therapeutic process of systemic constellations in more detail, certain "subprocesses" that contribute to the therapeutic effect can be identified. In direct relation to the client these are the following:

- Acquiring new knowledge;
- Realizing and expressing suppressed feelings;
- Fostering internal integration;
- Restoring the bond of love;
- Changing inner attitude.

Whereas considering the impact on the system, during constellations we deal with the following:

- Expression of trauma, abandonment, and pain of other members of the family;
- Establishing interrupted bonds between members of the family;

- Showing family secrets;
- Harmonization of the system in accordance with the orders of love.

The constellation provides new knowledge, showing roots of problems. It shows, for example, that the mother's brittleness did not result from the fact that she "did not love" her child, but from the fact that she was internally tied with someone, for example, with her sibling who died early, or carried someone's trauma. The new knowledge changes the perspective and is helpful in dealing with pain, grievance, or difficulty in accepting the parent. The knowledge is particularly important in constellations that address business or functioning of organizations. The client becomes aware, for example, of the indecisiveness of the potential business partner or the burden that he could bring to their joint undertaking, or notices the important condition for the success of the undertaking, which he did not take into account before.

The second factor concerns emotions and feelings. Constellations make it possible to express feelings, such as grievance, sense of guilt, or anger. It is possible to confront the suppressed feeling of loss and incomplete mourning. This happens not only in the usual form. Thanks to the fact that the client can be represented by another person, we reach emotions so deeply hidden that he would not be able to confront them himself. These processes are much more transformative than an ordinary abreaction. When the representative immerses himself in these difficult emotions, such as childlike fear, loneliness, anger, or pain, which are present in the client, the client himself immediately feels better.

The internal integration is described below and the changes in the inner attitude are analyzed in chapter 2. The restoration of the bond of love takes place when the individual opens up again or for the first time to his mother, father, siblings, and other people in his system. These bonds have always existed, but until now they have been hidden and unconscious, often causing life or health problems.

Let us now address the systemic level. The constellation does not only affect the individual's mind but also the family system he is connected with. Constellations have shown that a family system is not just a given group of people forming a family. The family system—the one we work with in constellations—is a certain energy and information matrix, in which all of us are immersed. The constellation affects precisely this matrix, which translates into the client's psychophysical state and can affect the persons who are just represented during the constellation.

The latter happens when the constellation concerns a child. The child is absent during the session, knows nothing about it, and yet feels its effects. One could give a number of examples that such sessions result in significant improvements in children's health or behavior.

Hence the unexpected changes in the attitudes of the loved ones and improbable "coincidences" so often reported by clients and constellation therapists. In the evening after the constellation, the client's mother calls her and says she has a gift for her, although she neither called nor gave her presents before. The day after the constellation, the client's eighty-year-old father says he will go for his birth certificate—it turns out that he was adopted, which explained the unclear aspects of the constellation. When the client returns from the constellation session, her mother spontaneously hugs her, for the first time in many years. The brother, who has not been heard from for several years, calls. The woman meets, for the first time, her husband's ex-wife, who played an important role in the constellation the day before. Such examples could be multiplied.

As therapists, clients and representatives, we do not have to understand everything that happened in the constellation. The process itself brings change. During the process, pain, fear, horror, loneliness, disgust, and humiliation—as if frozen in the family field—are released. The emotions experienced by the older members of the family, which they did not cope with and which became a burdening legacy for the younger ones. Bringing these experiences to light, together with the elements of the events they concern, in a way clears the client's system and is a kind of collective *catharsis*.

Uncovering family secrets, even though we cannot know them in detail, works in the same way. That is how they cease to be a terrible burden, which sometimes leads to the complete destruction of those who are born later. Such secrets often include the issues of paternity, adoption, former relationships and children, murders, and suicides.

The most important thing is that the constellation brings about the orders of love in the system. Someone's parents can find their way to their own parents; the early deceased or aborted children are remembered and accepted into the family; the perpetrators find their way to the victims. Of course, questions arise. What does it mean that the parents find their way to their parents and accept them into their hearts if they never did so before they died? What does it mean that the father in the constellation finally stopped confusing his daughter with his mother, if the "real" one has never changed anything in his behavior? The fact remains that these processes are deeply transformative. They are not an illusion or a fantasy. These transformations of systemic reality have a lasting effect on the client, and sometimes also change the attitudes of other people who were represented in the constellation, although they were physically absent. It can be said that the constellation brings out what is potential or hidden in the psyche of the system members. For example, the mother's love which could never break through her own problems and deficits. It is not imagined. It is true.

Changes take place in two parallel ways: as a result of conscious involvement and unconsciously. The conscious change happens already during the session, when the client observes the constellation and works on his own attitude, which requires conscious involvement (e.g., slow opening up to the parents, despite demotivating childhood events). He feels the changes on this plane directly and immediately—they take the form of a sense of unburdening, calmness, acceptance, a feeling of opening up internally, and inflow of energy. However, the constellation affects the client also without action on his part, if he—as Hellinger said—lets the picture of resolution get into his soul. This type of impact on the client develops gradually and can be extended over a period of two to three years.

THE MOVE IS UP TO THE CHILD

One may wonder to what extent the activity of the subject is essential in the process of development of disorders and to what extent these mechanisms are automatic and take place completely independently of any choices and internal decisions. Both internal, psychological in the narrower sense, as well as external systemic factors take part in the development of disorders. The first ones may be more or less dependent on the subject's will, but they must not be considered as fully conscious. If someone rejects his father, being completely indifferent to him, then this is a situation he has influence on—he could change his attitude toward his father. However, the reasons for this attitude are beyond the subject's will, they lie in the events of his childhood or in his mother's behavior. So currently, his influence on his own attitude toward his father turns out to be negligible, because the internal mechanisms shaped by the history of his life and environment consolidate his attitude.

So what happened completely unconsciously and regardless of our will gets incorporated through introjection in the sphere of our ego. Originally, it was something strange to us, now we begin to perceive it as our "choice," "character," "conscious decision," and "reasonable solution." This is how we see our conflicts with siblings, isolation from the mother, not talking to the father, or other things, such as living with the parents for too long or not working. Even if these are negative factors for us, we start to defend them, because we know nothing else. In this way, we sustain our own problems. But are we aware of this? No. Are we responsible for it? This is where things get complicated. Since we are not even aware of the origin of our attitudes, we cannot be responsible for them. On the other hand, there is no one else who could change something except ourselves.

Ultimately, it is us who are responsible for what happens to us. Hellinger writes that as a result of the early separation from the mother:

> Instead of approaching her with love, we rather stay away from her. The pain of early separation is too deep. And the other way round, if then the mother wants to approach the child with love and show and give him more of her love, the child often keeps away from her and rejects her. Here the mother's love for her child becomes largely powerless. (Hellinger 2014b, 47)[1]

This moment is well visible in constellations. The mother—that is, her representative—is open to the child—the client, she can and wants to give him, but the child cannot or does not want to open to it. The client, who stands in front of the representative of his mother, starts to remember the moments when the mother was inaccessible. These memories and the distrust and fear that he may again be rejected or ignored stop him from taking a step toward his mother. Usually, however, in the end, he succeeds, and even if not, the hidden desire to do so is activated.

Systemic constellations have discovered the power of unconscious factors that are independent from us, but they have also shown a great range of our agency. This is important in the context of extrication of oneself from childhood traumas, abandonment of suicidal tendencies, taking responsibility for one's own life, reconciliation with parents, and regaining the sense of vitality. Whether we take life and strength that flows to us depends on us. We are not so determined, marked, and dependent on the circumstances, as we often think. Even the idea of "changing the past" is not as absurd as it seemed. Until now, in psychotherapy, it looked different, for example, Alexander Lowen, referring to children separated from their mothers, who want to return to her their entire life, writes:

> But if the separation is definitive, the original connection cannot be restored any more than a fruit can be reattached to the tree. No matter how strenuous the attempt, it is destined to failure. This is the dilemma of the oral personality and it explains his predisposition to depression. (Lowen 1974, 57)

Many people wait in vain for the mother to change, show them warmth and love. But the author is wrong in thinking that it is impossible to restore the original bond. It is fully possible because it does not depend on the mother's attitude at all. Some people think they still need this or that from their mother, they are waiting for warm words, a hug, maybe some praise, or maybe for the mother to stop complaining, they think that then their lives would change for the better. They are right when they think that a good relationship with their mother is important for their well-being. However, they do not have to wait for their mother's move.

Your mother's attitude does not preclude you from getting from her what you need. For what you need is a connection to life and gratitude for it. And this is just up to you. You do not need—as much as you think—those expressions of love that manifest through your mother's behavior. What you need above all is to open up to the flow of life and strength, and these flow from your mother anyway. This flow may be blocked, but it does not disappear.

This completely new view of therapy results from the discovery of previously unknown processes. First, our parents are constantly present for us, regardless of whether we have contact with them and whether they live or not. Second, we ourselves remain, in a sense, a child. Third, as I mentioned above, there is a kind of life "energy" associated with the transmission of life from generation to generation. Opening up to this "energy" of our ancestors, flowing through our parents, turns out to be more important for our well-being from what we define as "feelings" or "warmth" on the part of the parents. To sum up, we have already received what we expect from our parents. It is life.

These facts show that radical changes in the area of our "tough childhood" are possible. People who did not get enough attention from their parents can get something from and through them that turns out to be more important than what they allegedly or actually lost. At the same time, this can be the beginning and the basis for changing the emotional attitude to our parents and the mutual relations.

As children, we reacted in a way that is common in children—when there were some difficulties in accessing the parent or when the parent failed our expectations, we closed in with our anger and resentment. As adults, when we face a representative of the parent, we are both the present ourselves and that child. Now, however, we know that it is up to us whether we will restore the bond between ourselves and the parent. The move is up to us. When this bond is rebuilt, the past begins to look different or we even have an impression of a retroactive influence on our childhood.

When we open ourselves to taking from our parents, we always get, there is always something to take (although this may require a longer process and working through transgenerational issues). When we finally take, we discover that as much as we got from them is enough. Feeling that the move is up to us, we free ourselves from the unfulfilled expectation and we see that we have already received from our parents everything that matters most. Hellinger writes about the bond with the mother:

> The first step comes from the child who, despite the pain of separation, again takes the first steps towards his mother. How can one start to take these steps? The child goes in his memory back to the time before that separation experience and imagines that he is taking the first small steps towards the mother, just as he naturally did before the separation. Now, as an adult child, he again takes a few steps towards the mother, with primal love, step by step, often for a long time, closer and closer to her. (Hellinger 2014b, 48)[2]

ACCEPTING THE MOTHER, ACCEPTING LIFE

Therapy of the early bond with the mother (and father), which we can conduct through constellations, uses similar processes to those addressed in Martha G. Welch's holding time method and Jirina Prekop's method of reconciliation with parents. While Welch's method is based on the work of the real parent with the child, Prekop uses substitutes too. Hellinger worked in a similar way; he became a representative of the parent and held the client, enabling him to express the pain of separation and patiently waiting for the movement of love to be restored. The direction of the process is always the same. The client's whole body and psyche, despite possible resistance, strives to reconstruct the bond.

Someone whose natural movement toward the mother was interrupted may initially jib at taking her into the heart, wanting to remain a rancorous child forever. Why? Because the loss of the mother is so great that it is hard to imagine getting out of it. But once they accept the connection to the mother, they feel the life flowing from her to them.

Reconstructing the early bond is important when someone was separated from their mother in childhood, had a particularly tough birth, or was born by caesarean section. Also when the mother died early, the bond with her is usually disrupted. Although at a deeper level, the psyche demands that this bond exist, the consciousness remains indifferent or even turns away from the memories of the mother. In someone who experienced the early death of his mother, there is a small child's anger that his mother died and left him. After all, a mother can do anything and if she dies, she does it because she is "bad." The child that internally turns away from the mother consequently turns away from life and becomes more susceptible to diseases.

When the client slowly approaches his mother, I often ask the child to open his hands with the palms turned upwards, and the mother to put her hands on them. Along with the process of internal opening up to the mother and leaving his mental pain, the client begins to clearly feel the flow of energy. It has nothing in common with bioenergy therapy, because the process is regulated purely psychologically, so it occurs only when the client is ready to emotionally open to the mother. However, what "flows" is something real, and in any case, it is a sign that one really opens up to the mother. Most importantly, the effects of such an opening are not limited to the possible improvement of someone's relationship with the mother. They are much more far-reaching—they are indicative of becoming open to life and health.

Accepting the mother is closely related to accepting life. As I wrote above, not accepting one's own life is very often connected with the perinatal period. This is when the child may distance himself from his mother for the first time, which will have significant consequences for his later life. In such a case, I ask the client to lie down on his side, in a fetal position. Then I represent his mother. Usually, the distance between the child and the mother is immediately apparent. It is in such cases that I sometimes set up one's "birth," as a representation of an important event that has determined the relationship between the mother and the child. Another time, I set up the father, as the one who initially welcomed the child when the mother was unable to do so, for example, due to postnatal depression. If the mother's relationship with her mother was disrupted, the latter may also be relevant here.

However, representing "life" often turns out to be most helpful. Many clients who experienced an interruption in their early relationship reject their own life. It is difficult for them to look at the person who represents it; they say that they do not want their life, that life disappointed them, and so on. Only in the therapeutic situation, where life is "personified," do they realize that they reject what constitutes them on such a fundamental level. Most clients are, however, able to overcome their aversion to life, realizing that there is no other constructive attitude than accepting their own life, as it is together with the context in which it came to us.

Helping one accept one's life, one's mother, one's parents, or acknowledge the hierarchy is possible and feasible in a relatively short time because there are attractors that lead us in this direction. It is not that we have to strongly convince clients that they should give up this or that attitude and adopt a different one, because it will prove to be better for them. The people present in the constellation session realize and start to feel what is right themselves. Here we have the interaction of the family field and, as we could call it, the client's true self. The family field manifested during the constellation shows what forces influence the individual and what place is right for him. The true self, that is, for example, the sincere childlike part of the client, shows him that he is still attached to his mother and needs from her "what the mother gives," that is, the flow of life-love. By standing in this flow, he places himself in the broad current of life that reaches far into the past. Only in this way, by going beyond one's individual organism toward the life of the family, can one remain healthy.

RECONCILIATION WITH PARENTS AND THE ENERGY OF ANCESTORS

Those who regret that they have a bad relationship with their parents are often closer to mental health than those for whom it is not a problem. Even before I got acquainted with constellations, when conducting psychotherapy, I observed that there seemed to be something inhuman about those who excluded one of their parents. The more the father or mother was unimportant to them, nonexistent, indifferent, or somehow unwelcome, the more those people acted mechanically, were in some measure desensitized, as if partially deprived of what is the most human. Sometimes they seemed as if they lost their minds or were intellectually limited. They lacked some flexibility and emotional understanding. When in the course of psychotherapy, they were able to open to the fact of the existence and meaning of the parent, they started to be perceived as multidimensional and more human. Later, when I got to know constellations, the phenomenon became clearer to me.

Suggesting reconciliation with parents, that is, accepting "parents as parents," is not a moral recommendation, but arises from the recognition of one of the basic needs of the psyche. At a deeper level, the psyche always demands that we be emotionally connected to those through whom we have come into the world. The fact that our parents are the beginning of our lives is an existential truth. It turns out that this fact—that we are flesh and blood of the mother and father—has far-reaching consequences and cannot, for our sake, be ignored. It is difficult for some people to see this, because they think of themselves as if they were always here, always decided about themselves. This unconscious memory demands to be acknowledged and moved to the conscious level. This is what the acceptance of our "parents as parents," as the biological beginning of ourselves, is.

There may be a doubt regarding the acceptance of parents. One could think that some parents are so bad for their child that they should be rejected by him. But can a child do it without harming himself? The psychic level that we address here demands accepting parents, regardless of how they behaved. If for some reason it did not happen, problems will arise.

Of course, children did not fabricate their difficulties in accepting their mother or father. Even if the image of their parents is not accurate, early abandonment, emotional absence, psychological problems of the parent, alcoholism, and so on underlie it. However, these also usually have a transgenerational background, and constellations enable one to see and understand it all, and thus enable the client to approach even the parent he rejected before.

Through accepting the parents, we can open up for acceptance of the energy of the ancestors, and this is the acceptance of life as something flowing from afar. There is nothing metaphorical or related to faith here, but real and perceptible processes. When, open to our parents, we stand at the top of our family pyramid, with our parents, grandparents, and great-grandparents behind us, we will feel a distinct flow of energy. This is not an ephemeral phenomenon, but it brings positive effects for good. In this way, we root ourselves, stabilize our own identity, calm down, and find strength for life's tasks.

Brayden said he had a problem with his own identity, self-esteem, and confidence. When he walked on the sidewalk, he thought to himself that the man walking from the opposite direction was "a psychopath" and would attack him in a moment. This kind of thinking ruined his life. In the constellation, his father, who had difficulty accepting his own father, was important. Brayden's father was attached to his mother and despised his own father. Both of them—the client's representative and his father's representative—stood in the constellation, embracing their mothers, as if taking their fathers' places. It was only when the representative of Brayden's father lay down in front of his father and acknowledged the hierarchy that Brayden could look at him with more respect. When finally he stood in the men's line in person and opened up to the strength flowing from it, he experienced very intense feelings. It was unusual and surprising to him that the experience was so clear and strengthening.

When a man stands in the generational string, he has his father, grandfather, then his great-grandfather, and sometimes the great-great-grandfather behind his back. Then he takes masculine strength and energy through them. Behind a woman's back there is her mother and other ancestresses from whom she takes the same. It is a transgenerational transmission of masculine and feminine strength that makes it possible for us to be a man or a woman in a better way. Whatever the nature of this energy, we clearly feel it and intuitively understand it. Opening oneself up to it and taking one's place with respect in this generational current gives one the feeling of greater rooting and stability. The impact of this procedure—like of most other procedures in constellations—is not limited to just soothing or vital feelings. We can stand in the generational string after some work, when we are ready to take this place. Taking the right place in the constellation is also taking the right place in our own life. The feeling of being in the "right place," the sense of strength and the connection with the ancestors result in better abilities to cope in the world.

GOING BEYOND THE OLD NARRATIONS

Distancing oneself from burdensome memories is a positive change factor. Many people carry them within themselves as lasting and outwardly coherent narrations that are supposed to explain their lives and failures. It is amazing how often these stories are banal. However, we are often absolutely sure that they are of fundamental meaning. One woman said quite seriously that she had been hurt by her mother who had praised her sister's dress and had "just looked at her." These types of stories are told as traumatic events that have governed a person's life, for example, by depriving them of their self-esteem. The most important thing is the words that are spoken in such situations, starting with, for instance: "Follow your brother's example," "You're not suitable for this," "You're unbearable," and ending with: "I regret I gave birth to you." Although sentences of the last type can be extremely hurtful, it is us who make them really strong. They are not so significant as such, and generally, if not always, they do not express the parent's true and only attitude. Nor do they eliminate love.

How do we go beyond these narrations in constellations? By accepting people and at the same time leaving the events associated with them. Sometimes I simply say to the client, "Now you are leaving these memories. These things happened, but now you don't think about them. You are only looking at your father and accepting him as your father. You don't think about anything else." It has nothing to do with denying reality. The point is to open up to contact with the parent as a parent. This process is much more important than the events remembered.

If a woman's grandfather spoke ill of her and was unpleasant, she accepts him as her grandfather, "leaving his words with him." Constellations show that such a procedure is not imaginative; it is not a kind of suggestion and programming of one's mind. The grandfather can indeed be accepted, and this acceptance radically increases the ability to detach oneself from what was negative about the relationship with him. I define it as a double move—accepting someone as a person makes it possible to leave what binds us to him in a negative way. Of course, this process primarily concerns the people with whom we are systemically most connected, such as our parents, grandparents, and siblings. It is in our relationships with them that it is best seen that one cannot free oneself from negative influences of the past unless the bond is acknowledged.

In Briana's constellation, her mother's representative felt that she hated her daughter and wanted to kill her. Briana was not at all surprised—the picture corresponded to what she experienced from her mentally ill mother. As Briana said, her mother did not beat her but tortured her. Briana also remembered her father abusing her sexually. What the mother experienced in the constellation was a kind of madness; the great-grandmother was in a similar state. Two or three generations of women in their family experienced this "murderous madness," which was rooted in the war. The senseless killing of the loved ones and friends affected the great-grandmother, grandmother, and other family members, and was more than they could mentally endure. A kind of untroubled desire to kill experienced by Briana's great-grandmother and mother (the representative of one of them said she wanted to "experiment" killing) seemed to be a defense mechanism, a kind of internal coping with the trauma. It was suppressed but manifested itself through their uncontrollable and aggressive behaviors.

What brought the solution was adding a representative of the war. The mother and great-grandmother regained mental balance. The madness slowly left them. Their "deadliness" could not overcome the power of war and trauma. Eventually, Briana began to feel more and saw her mother as a mother, which had been very difficult for her before. Before that, all she had was her traumatic story of a child who had not had a childhood and who had "taken care of her mother" from an early age. Now the mother stopped being insane and could give to the daughter. Was the mother's "sanity" an artificial product of the constellation? No, it was hidden in her, buried under the transgenerational trauma. Now, after going beyond the old stories and victim identity, Briana could start taking from her mother.

We all create our autobiographies—more or less coherent stories of our own lives and the most important events in them. In general, the ideas we have about our fates do not show much psychological complexity. Even psychologists who avidly publish their ideas about the causes of human problems and behaviors in magazines and books support us in building these simplified patterns. For example, the father's alcoholism makes it easy to explain many aspects of one's own life. How many people "know" that their failures, relationship problems, and difficulties with themselves are due to the fact that their "father was a drunk"? You can throw everything that is wrong in our lives into the father's bottle. When they hear that "alcohol was abused at home," many therapists seem to have got to the heart of the problem.

Constellations make it possible to go beyond the simplistic stories with which we try to explain our whole reality. It is especially important to go beyond other people's stories—often heard from mothers. A constellation enables one to separate oneself and one's opinion from that of others. For instance, it is generally difficult for an alcoholic's adult child to look at his father and recognize his relationship with him. A constellation makes it possible for him to separate the father from his alcoholism. He can see the background of the father's problems, which is sometimes love for someone from the family. This kind of relativization of the alcohol problem liberates the child. He gets the father back and at the same time breaks with the mother's judgments and opinions. Thus, he gains greater internal autonomy.

One of my clients, Veronica, told me that when she was four, her father "jumped out of his car and stuffed a toy under her arm." She was terrified and threw the toy away. Even when she told me about it, she seemed to be referring to it as a villain's attack. This is how the child, whose eyes were controlled by her mother, saw it. In fact, the father simply gave her a gift, taking advantage of the fact that he met her, as the mother prevented his contact with the daughter. In adulthood, of course, she could not function with men in a normal way, she idealized them and demanded too much from them or devaluated them. When a child separates his view from that of his mother, he becomes individualized. He begins to see his father differently, but he also sees the mother differently. The mother may lose her "holiness" and "heroism." There may be a grievance against her. If this happens, it does not have to be anything bad—this is a stage in becoming aware and mature.

TRANSGENERATIONAL CONSCIOUSNESS

Many people believe that the root of their problems lies in their childhood experiences, and point to their parents as the main wrongdoers. The parents' actions and words are said to have had a decisive influence on the difficulties in their lives. From this perspective, the parents become the only rulers and administrators of these lives. Of course, it is impossible to negate their role in the development of the child, but in this way, they are denied their humanity, they become like gods. The truth about man's mental development is completely different—life is influenced by a wide systemic context. Our parents are a part of it, and our fate may be determined by an unconscious relationship with someone we have not even heard of. When we look at the parents, we tend to see them isolated; we do not see what determined them. Thanks to constellations, the parents cease to be the rulers of our lives because they are relativized—we see that they too are people and children of their parents. This broadens our view of our own lives and enables us to breathe deeper.

Emily said she "realized that she had always been a victim" of her mother first, then of her husband. The mother was attached to religious norms, she was intrusive and suppressed her daughter's spontaneity and sexuality, and at the same time she was suffering, hesitant, she expected support, which resulted in the reversal of caring roles. Without a doubt, Emily was burdened by her mother, but did she know what this burden really was? When I stood as the mother, I immediately began to look for something. I took a watering can and put it on the floor, cringing close to it. Emily remembered that her mother said there was something "she wouldn't say," a secret. At the same time, she felt relieved, better. I realized that the secret was represented by the bottle. After a while the client said that "it was something sexual" (I also had a thought that there was something phallic about the bottle, but I did not share it).

When I stood as the grandmother, I understood that the relationship between Emily's mother and her mother was the same as the one between Emily and her mother. I felt as if I wanted to hide something, ordered silence and self-restraint, perhaps as if I could not accept a stain on the family's honor. Finally, as the grandmother, I stood with the grandfather represented by another object. It turned out that what the bottle symbolized was their business. Emily and her mother had to leave it with them.

The confusing and burdening "sexual mystery" was uncovered. It did not have to be defined exactly (I guessed that the grandfather might have sexually abused Emily's mother, but I could not be sure of that and did not mention it). However, the constellation made it possible to see the mother in a new light—she too was a victim of what was happening in the family. She transmitted, not generated the problem.

In this way, we can also help adopted people who do not know their biological parents. Some of them are unable to find out the truth about their ancestry or meet the living family members. They feel sad and are emotionally instable. Thanks to constellations, they can become aware of their own roots. They can touch the fate of their real parents and better understand their own fate. Those who do not know their parents will not get answers to specific questions about their identity through constellations, but they can astonishingly clearly show the context in which the child was given up for adoption. Sometimes the picture that emerges during the constellation suggests that the child was given away in good faith, that this is how the parent understood what would be good for the child. The client also sees his grandparents and even great-grandparents, which widens his sense of identity. In this broader context, the individual becomes stronger.

Transgenerational awareness as an element of therapy can be found, for example, in the exercises proposed by Prekop as part of her School of Love in the Family. The therapist proposes a visualization during which we imagine the family home and ourselves as children and recollect the pain our father or mother caused us. Then, from an adult position, we visualize our parent as a child. The author writes:

> So you are looking with your adult eyes at your mother (father) and her (his) childhood. Let this image come to you. You see the child who later became your mother (father) and her (his) pain. How old is the child? How is she (he) dressed? Is there anyone with her (him) or is she (he) all alone? What is she (he) looking at? What are her (his) hands doing? When you realize the child's misery, tell her (him), "I understand you. It's tough for you." (Prekop 2015, 56)[3]

It happens that a father leaves his family and does not want to keep in contact with his child. Constellations create an opportunity to see such an event from a wider perspective. It may turn out that the father is attached to his mother, who died when he was just a few years old. Then what determines his step in the first place is not his attitude toward his child's mother, let alone toward the child, but the bond with his own mother. In addition, seeing that he remained a child inside himself because the broken bond made it impossible for him to fully mature, it is easier to understand his limited ability to fully assume the role of a parent. Of course, he remains a father and the child needs to accept him as a father, and this turns out to be more possible after he sees the above context.

UNBURDENING AND RETURNING TO ONESELF

Leaving What Is Not Ours

One of the most important processes in constellations is giving back to others or leaving in the past what is not ours. For we can carry somebody else's fate, somebody else's affairs, traumas, and guilts, or subconsciously experience past injustices. This causes us to separate from ourselves internally. Our life energy dies, and everything becomes much more difficult. Alienation can manifest itself in such a way that in the constellation, we see ourselves in the representative of the deceased person rather than our own. What then are our own body, life, and relationships that we enter into? It is tough for us, because in a sense we are not present. By resolving the entanglement, we slowly stop looking internally at another person. Then we can look at our own lives.

We are most strongly alienated by the entanglement with the people who died before we were born and who we have never met in person. Then everything happens completely unconsciously. There are, however, alienating processes that involve the relationships with the living, especially with parents. The mother may see the child who died earlier in her living child. The father may see his ex-partner in his daughter. The children raised in such dynamics will be constantly influenced by their parents' projections. And they will respond to them, they will usually obey them. Thus, they may face gender identity problems if the deceased sibling was of the opposite sex, or difficulties in romantic relationships if they assume the role of the father's partner.

However, even if the mother or father still projects their problems onto us, we can decide not to carry them any longer. It is our right to take our lives from our parents, and leave their unresolved issues and guilt with them. Regardless of the bond and love, we say, "You for yourself, I for myself." This is particularly important when our loyalty to the parents pushes us toward death or blocks us from going into our own lives.

A child wants to take depression, grief, mourning off his parent, and stop his pursuit of death. Sometimes he wants to save someone in his great-grandparents' generation. Or share his father's guilt. All these are burdens that he unwittingly, but willingly, takes on himself. "Taking" from past generations may seem abstract or metaphorical. It is different. Constellations show that it is something that has a real impact on man's life. We can see that "taking" is real also because "giving back" during a constellation is a psychophysical experience. When we leave in the past what belongs to the past, what we unconsciously got involved in, we feel real physical unburdening.

We can "leave" the burdens rooted in the distant past, which we were not aware of, as well as those we experienced consciously. For instance, someone feels burdened by their relationship with their mother because they feel guilty every time they leave her house. But bringing the mother's parents in the constellation immediately causes relief—it becomes clear that the mother internally has not come to terms with their death, and her sense of being "abandoned" is related to them, not to her child.

For several decades, Eliza felt anxiety in social situations. She often felt, for example, when doing the shopping in a supermarket, that other people could hurt her. These emotional states caused her to isolate herself and not do many things. In the constellation, an important thread was something "murderous" related to the grandmother. In this constellation, the client, once she was aware of this material, could express her intention to leave it in the past. As experience shows, such an internal, conscious intention (complemented, for example, by bowing to the representations of the ancestors) has a transformative and lasting effect.

When Eliza came again two months later, she said her old fears disappeared. This time she wanted to work on the relationship with her father. Her father had "always" been sick, complained about a variety of maladies, and was currently in a relationship with a doctor (the client thought it was primarily because she looked after him). He often called her, instructed her, told her what to do. After such a call, she was unstable, nervous, and it worsened her relationship with her husband.

When I stood as the father, I asked the client how she felt. She replied she felt nothing, she was like frozen. Later in the session, she felt as if something was pulling her back, further away from her father. As the father's representative, I understood that there was something heavy he was bound to. I intuitively felt that it concerned his mother. I put an object on the floor as his mother. I felt a strange state of psychic pain, bordering on insanity, which indicated a disturbed bond, probably in the perinatal period. After some time, I finally felt calm, touching the object representing the mother. Then I said to the client, "I mistook you for someone else," "You're just a child," "Now I see you as my daughter." Then Eliza could approach her father and hug him. That made it possible for her to get closer to her husband, who was also represented in the constellation.

This case illustrates the father's projection and the child's response to it. In such a situation both of them have a problem. The child—because she cannot adequately respond to the parent's unconscious demands and becomes tied down with them. The father—because he cannot reach his mother, as it seems to him that he could get what he needs from his daughter.

Eve underwent five years of psychotherapy, and now she suffered a nervous breakdown and had suicidal thoughts. As she said, the reason for her condition was the behavior of her partner, who entered into various relationships with other women. She said that she had "worked through a lot," but during the conversation, it became clear that she had not resolved the basic issues. She was not reconciled with her mother; she did not accept her father, with whom she had no contact. An important moment of her constellation (with figurines) was the difficulty for Eve's mother to accept her mother. At first, when I asked "what she felt," pointing to the mother figurine, Eve either answered that she did not know or said with a noticeable aversion, "She feels nothing, she has never felt anything." I did not comment on it, admitting everything that came from the client.

Eve began to notice her mother's resentment toward her own mother. It did not contradict what she remembered from her life. I was aware that Eve's attitude toward her mother was exactly the same, but I did not refer to it at all. Eve, concentrated on the figurines, said that she was all moved and felt confused. At the end, discovering some orders by herself, such as a bow, she accepted her life as a gift from her parents. She also asked if she could accept "only this"—as if not trusting the parents completely and being afraid of the burdens associated with them. I said "Yes, because this is the most important thing."

Internal Integration

In constellations, we often observe dissociation within the client's psyche. Certain aspects of the self, usually related to early painful feelings or later traumas, are cut off and deeply buried. Constellations make it possible for one to reintegrate internally, thus regain the lost mental energy. The split-off part of the psyche can be represented by the therapist or another person, then the client concentrates on his reactions to this part of himself. It is a common occurrence that the client at first rejects the split-off part. For this "part" of himself is usually full of fear, crying, and lonely. It is the memory of childhood pain and helplessness; it is actually the child he once was. A constellation reveals, with incredible clarity, the mechanisms of keeping those painful aspects of oneself away from consciousness. Often, clients are extremely insensitive to their "inner child" in the beginning, as if they were afraid that by getting closer to it they will weaken. However, agreeing to it and accepting it as an inseparable part of themselves is the way to regaining mental strength and not losing it. When in the course of the constellation, the client approaches the representative of his inner child, embraces him or only touches him, and at the same time, he stops defending himself against the recognition that all these emotions exist in him. He then feels that he is becoming more complete and understands himself better.

Paul caused an accident in which two young men died and one person became an invalid. When he concentrated on a device in his car for a moment, he pulled into the opposite lane, causing that two other cars crashed. The client already had two constellations—both led us to the people who died and showed his guilty feeling. He came to the next constellation, saying that he did not use his intuition, his resources, and that he could not make important decisions. I guessed what he could be talking about, and Paul confirmed my assumptions, saying that he felt as if he "wasn't fully there."

I asked him to put a piece of paper on the floor representing that "part" of him that was separate. I stood as the representative of that part. Paul looked at my shoes, felt various physical symptoms, but could not raise his eyes or make a step. Later, he said that my hands caught his attention, which he associated with his father's work-worn hands. Later in the process, I felt that someone else also mattered here—as the "part of him," I looked at someone from the side. I set up an object in that place, and then I started to represent that person. My eyes immediately fell on the word "kill" in the title of one of the books in my office. As the person I represented, I began to rub my hands in a characteristic way, which indicated actions that caused a sense of guilt. I asked if there were any events related to sudden or dramatic deaths in his family. Paul immediately replied that it was his grandfather who had served in the Wehrmacht.

Paul was separated from the part of his soul that was connected to his grandfather and his family in general. In this way, he reacted to the trauma of the accident and the unconscious thought that he was repeating some pattern associated with death and hard lot (during the constellation he also mentioned two of his relatives who died in the World War I). Now slowly and with fear, he integrated with the cut-off part and through it with his family system. He now felt the strength within him and said that he was standing on his feet more firmly.

In cases where we deal with sexual harassment, the greatest trauma for the child—as constellations show—is the loss of his family niche, his relationship with the mother in particular. It is difficult for the child to continue to feel like a child and to turn to his mother. He feels guilty, strange, and detached. In such cases, the traumatized part of the psyche is split off. If the therapist stands as this part, for example, the six-year-old girl who was molested, then usually the client initially rejects the split-off part. However, accepting this part is a fundamental step toward transcending the trauma and moving toward internal reintegration. In this case, when trying to make the client accept her own childlike part, we also work with her to rebuild the bond with her mother. These two processes are interdependent.

A Good Balance

A participant of my constellation training course, Blanca, during her own work, complained about her fear of driving. This made her life difficult, as her profession required frequent traveling. She was conceived, as she said, in a car—by a driving instructor who taught her mother. She already had a husband, but after she got pregnant, she got divorced. Blanca had no contact with her father, they did not meet. Her relationship with the mother was difficult. I set up representatives of Blanca, her mother, her mother's ex-husband, and her biological father. The representative of Blanca's mother panicked in this constellation, she was extremely afraid of her ex-husband, she wanted him to say something, but he did not respond. At the same time, she talked about a great desire to have sex, to be "fucked." The biological father was angry and felt used. Blanca's representative stood in front of the mother's ex-husband from the beginning. Further in the constellation, Blanca's mother told her ex-husband to confess something, to reveal something, she felt despised by him, she said that this was why "his penis didn't work." At the same time, she pointed to Blanca's father, calling him a "real alpha male." Blanca's representative stood fixedly in front of her mother's ex-husband, feeling particularly attached to him.

After some time, it became clear for everyone that the ex-husband really kept something secret, perhaps some events related to sexual violence in his family (which manifested itself thanks to another representative). The representatives had the impression that somehow his manipulations and hiding the truth—from himself and others—contributed to the subsequent course of events. As if he passively pushed his wife into the arms of another man.

When Blanca was brought in the constellation in person, she also clearly felt connected to the representative of her mother's ex-husband. What made her so strongly bound to him? What inner gesture and what words could enable her to go into her life, and before to turn to her parents, who were so far indifferent to her? I finally understood what it was about. Blanca felt she lived thanks to the attitude of her mother's ex-husband. Thanks to the way he was, what he did, she came into the world. She stood by him as if she wanted to compensate him for the gift of her life. What was the solution? A conscious "Thank you" brought her a feeling of great relief.[4]

This constellation led to balance that was an unconscious need of the client. A similar need, although even stronger, is present in adopted people who did not have the opportunity to find out about their biological parents or for some reason—for instance, loyalty to their adoptive parents—to express their gratitude.

NOTES

1. Quotation translated from German.
2. Quotation translated from German.
3. Quotation translated from Polish.

4. This was still not enough for the client to be able to fully separate herself from this man. It was not until I brought in a representative, whom I defined as "something that all life comes from" and set this representative behind all the representatives that the situation changed. Blanca could now detach herself from the man and look at her parents. The biological father stopped feeling used and calmed down. Blanca approached her parents and cuddled up to them. She was no longer an "illegitimate child," as she had called herself, but her parents' child. Whose life, like the life of each of us, came from afar. And took many people into its service.

Part II

APPLICATION OF SYSTEMIC CONSTELLATIONS IN PSYCHOTHERAPY AND COACHING

Chapter 4

Relationships and Their Problems

RELATIONSHIP OF NOT JUST TWO

To love a partner is to give. If we feel that we should receive particularly much from our partner, if he is to protect us from the overwhelming feeling of loneliness, if we expect him to fill our whole life, being constantly with us without a moment for himself, and finally if we are jealous of his work, passion, or interpersonal contacts—he is not the point.

So who is the point in such cases? Very often it is the mother. Sometimes it is another person, but always someone from our family system—someone who has "accompanied" us since childhood, although we may have been completely unaware of it.

A woman in her forties, Olivia, told me during a workshop that she loved a man she had met as a child. She has a husband now, but that man appeared for a while in her life a few years ago, which broke her down. Is this unfulfilled great love? Yes, but completely different and for someone else. When we set up her representative and the man's representative, one could immediately feel that he was not the point. I realized I should ask about her relationship with the mother. It was not good, and the client had long since moved away from her mother. This absent, but living in her thoughts and emotions, man represented the distant and secretly loved mother. He had no other meaning. This may be an extreme case of "romantic" love, but every love choice is similar to it—Hellinger says that both men and women look for their mother in a relationship. The mother figure is central here, because it is the bond with her that is the matrix of all close relationships.

John felt he could not come to an understanding with his wife. He maintained that he was empathetic toward his children and that his wife was too harsh. He was focused on development, his wife was a traditionalist strongly attached to Christianity. He said all this made him withdraw and become an "observer."

I started the individual constellation by choosing four positions: John, "what he brings into the relationship with his wife," the wife, "what she brings into the relationship with him." When I stood as "what the wife brings into the relationship," I cowered, grabbed my stomach, and breathed quickly. This kind of feeling usually occurs when something difficult related to procreation and delivery is involved. While standing as the wife, I felt some kind of fear, uncertainty, and difficulty in looking at the husband. I asked John how he felt. He said he wanted to help his wife, take care of her.

Then I stood as "something that John brings into the relationship." From this position, I put my hands around his neck from behind, looking at the "wife" sheet over his shoulder. Then I approached the sheet and I spontaneously started to move as if I were stroking the wife, following her contours with my hands, focusing especially on her breasts. I felt a kind of love and adoration. I asked about his attitude toward his mother. John: "I worship my mother." Then I stood as the mother. She had a lot of love for her son. The client said that he always tried to deserve his mother's love. She was his teacher at school, in the first classes, and she was demanding.

What was important at that point? It was best for John to allow himself to simply take from his mother and leave the thought that he had to "deserve" it. When, after working on John's relationship with his mother, I stood as his wife again, I moved away from him at first. Why? I understood that his wife felt his inner change. But then, still as the wife, I looked at him and started approaching him. We stood for a while looking into each other's eyes. John felt more open to his wife now. She was also interested in him. The rest was up to them. What did this constellation result in? It made it possible to separate the wife from the mother—note that in John's childlike eyes she was also harsh and demanding. It pointed to the importance of loving his mother instead of "worshiping" her, which made it possible for him to put aside his need to "deserve" his mother's feeling. This will enable John to be his inner mother's child, a child that can take from her. This will help him to look at his wife in a different way and expect something different from her.

This does not mean that the father is unimportant. It may be that he is the one who will mark all relationships between a woman and her men. That was the case with Melanie. She was in a relationship with a man for seven years, and when it ended, she realized that she had completely neglected herself and lost her boundaries. That is why she then tried not to enter into erotic relationships. She wondered for a long time what she wanted, what kind of man. She came to a constellation session, saying that "now she wanted a relationship," but still hesitated and feared.

During our conversation, she mentioned that she had talked to a friend about constellations. The friend had two individual constellations with me, she also attended a training course and a workshop. Melanie said that such "continuation" and "long-term" frightened her. Once a therapist offered her therapy and said it was a serious commitment, and the client got frightened. I asked her what she was so scared of.

Melanie: "An addiction, losing myself, what I think."
Therapist: "That means you feel you have a tendency toward this."
M: "Yes."

I stood as the "potential man/the man in her life." I lowered my head, closed my legs, doubled over—I felt insecure and fearful.

T: "Do my attitude and feelings tell you anything?"
M: "It's my father."

I took an extra sheet of paper, wrote "father" on it, and then I stood on it as her father. Indeed, the dynamics were almost identical. Then I stood as her father's mother—here too, the movement and feelings were similar, which indicated that the son took something over from the grandmother. I stood as "the cause of what was happening to the father's mother." In this role, I grabbed myself by the throat as if I were suffocating and fell on the floor. Melanie had been sobbing for some time. Her grandmother and father were subconsciously tied to something difficult. I also represented the father's older brother who had committed suicide—he did not want to look at it all, he wanted to cut himself off, to move away, but he was also attached to it.

The client simply thanked her ancestors, by "giving back the past to the past." When I stood as the "man" again, I spontaneously stretched out my arms toward her, which was a sign that the systemic situation had changed. I was open and ready, everything now depended on her. What happened here? Melanie looked at her father, and without getting involved in his burdens, she could accept him more fully. In this way, the father and the potential man were separated, which Melanie felt very clearly. So now she no longer had to look for him in another man. This made her more ready for a relationship.

There is no recipe for a successful relationship. The intimate relationship does not have the same coherence and unambiguity as the partners' family of origin systems. While bringing the orders of love into the system results in a lasting improvement in our well-being and functioning, the relationship remains something dynamic. According to Hellinger, there is, however, a certain pattern of relationship between man and woman in which a marriage can be successful. The pattern is as follows: "The woman follows the man and the man serves the woman." In this arrangement, the issue of power struggle in the relationship is resolved—the woman follows the man. The issue of respect for the woman is also resolved—the man serves her. The pattern is basically to express the desires and natural abilities of both sexes: to be receptive and submissive for the woman, and to lead and protect for the man. It seems that although such an arrangement is not part of the strict orders of love, it will be functional in most cases. Nowadays, one tries not to notice that this division of roles corresponds to the deep emotional levels of many people. Instead, the principle of equal division of tasks is advocated, without paying attention to the fact that this proposal also demands an equal division of desires and abilities, and this does not seem possible.

Relationships last thanks to our efforts. However, neither man nor woman says, "I love you" only as individuals, "behind them stand the parents and the ancestors and the fates" (Hellinger 2008a, 28).[1] Some would like to avoid these efforts or taking into account the affairs of their ancestors. That is why they dream of "karmic relationships," "twin souls," and that people are "destined" for each other. These are all either illusions or the result of a longing for someone else—for example, the twin who died in the mother's womb. Constellations clearly show how much our relationships depend on the family of origin. In them we look for the issues and people belonging to our family.

However, people do not pair off randomly. There is unconscious perception behind it. We see in each other things that we do not know about on the conscious level, and they attract us to each other: a similar family situation, similar unconscious attitudes, or complementary things, opposite to ours. Sometimes one partner takes on himself the psychological problems of the other. For example, self-destructiveness and the move toward death. But it probably only happens when these dynamics correspond somehow to his own problems that started in his family of origin. In this respect, we can look at our partners as people who can teach us something about ourselves.

Since every relationship is created on the basis of the experience that we already had and that we project onto the people we meet, is it possible to love a given person, not one's own memories and unfulfilled desires? It is, but this love is always shaped by what we carry within us. Not only by what we experienced in our childhood, but also what we experience within ourselves now. Because my relationship with my mother or father depends not only on my childhood events but also on my current internal attitude toward my parents. I can change it and thus change my attitude toward my partner. However, I will not cut myself off from my roots, and if I try to do so, my relationship will turn out to be empty or my children will take over the problem. For we do not bring just ourselves into a relationship, we smuggle past baggage into it, often neatly wrapped and hidden. If we are reconciled with our family of origin and have resolved basic entanglements, we bring the people supporting us, our parents, grandparents, and great-grandparents in the relationship. Then our partner can lean on us, because we lean on our ancestors. If we are not reconciled with our family, if we harbor a grievance and anger, then problems enter into the relationship. From our misfortunate partner, one might say, we expect the impossible—solving them. Hence, the frequent arguments, reproaches, anger, and pain that we experience in our intimate relationships.

A woman may run away from her relationships with men and hide under her father's wing, thinking that no man is good enough for her. However, this happens only when the father is not fully accepted as a father. And when the daughter does not fully occupy the position of his child. Such a daughter tries to be her father's partner or the father wants to see her as his partner. Why does this happen? The father may see his ex-partner in the daughter, and she may gladly represent her. Only when the daughter stops playing this game and accepts the real position of the daughter will she be able to become more open to men.

It can be similar with a man who sticks to his mother. Does he love her so much? Possibly, but his love will take a more complete form when he accepts his mother as a mother and gives up her partner's position. Of course, there are mothers who like this situation. They often did not accept their father, and now they do not respect their son's father. Later, the son may be afraid of closeness with women. This condition is caused by the way the man experiences his mother. A mother is not a father. A woman is not a man. The mother is always more possessive and absorbing, that is part of her nature, or that is certainly how children see it. It is the mother's version of the family story that is most heard. It is the mothers who teach, heal, judge, speak a lot, feed, and take care. They are everywhere. Sometimes it is too much, especially for a boy. The more so because he pushes himself completely into his mother's arms. If the father does not intervene to drag the boy away from his mother, when he grows up and enters into a relationship with a woman, he will feel that it is "too much." He will experience his partner's every requirement as a burden and will try to avoid it, and even if there are no requirements, he will see them.

Hellinger says that most major conflicts between spouses result from a double shift. The spouses argue fiercely, while it is not about them and their affairs. One or both of the partners fight for things that are not theirs and with the wrong opponent. But that is why these wranglings over "socks" are so fierce—we can feel, as Hellinger says, so entitled only if we act in someone else's name and are unaware of the real reasons. A woman may be afraid of men and not trust them, and the reason may be the events in the distant past. Some man could have hurt, for example, raped, a woman from her family.

The woman will project this unconscious knowledge and trauma onto men, with whom she will be in relationships.[2]

Systemic constellations show that the determinants of the quality of the relationship and our feeling in it go far beyond the intimate relationship. After 20 years of her unsatisfactory relationship, Camilla discovered that she was a "victim." She also understood that she no longer wanted to be the victim. Her husband criticized her, treated her badly, and even beat her. The constellation revealed a surprising picture. It turned out that it was about her grandfather and many other people, perhaps about war-related matters. There was a blurred picture of many people and the dynamics of the grandfather's guilt. When I informed the client about it, she said that the grandfather was a soldier and executioner. Neither of us had thought that the problem with the husband would lead to such a source. So there were victims that Camilla, through her grandfather, identified with. In the constellation, she was afraid of her husband. This fear disappeared when she accepted her grandfather and bowed to the victims. She could now afford not to be one of them.

Malvina did not find common ground with her husband, who constantly criticized the fact that she "faffed around," that is, that she attended psychological trainings and additional studies in this field instead of doing something "concrete." The constellation revealed that the husband was particularly bound to someone. When I stood as that person, I moved in a strange way, as if I wanted to embrace something huge with my hands, I started to goggle and felt something "crazy." I asked Malvina if there were any mental disorders in her husband's family and she confirmed. The grandmother was said to be "not right in the head." The client's husband was very close to his grandmother. This bond resulted in his fear of madness, which was manifested in his disapproval of his wife's "psychological" interests and the fact that when they quarreled, no arguments spoke to him, and Malvina had the impression that her husband was a "madman." When I represented him in the constellation and took the grandmother into the heart, I could stop being afraid of madness, look at the wife differently, and accept her interests.

Ada said she could not stop her relationship that was "harmful for her." At the same time, she broke relationships that could be successful. She believed that the reason why she continued this pattern was the fact that her father "used violence." We could think it was a fairly good explanation and assume that she replicated the traumatic relationship with her father. However, in the constellation, her grandfather's mother turned out to matter here. She experienced some great trauma associated with her femininity, her child, maybe delivery. Her son was emotionally frozen and his relationship with his daughter (Ada's mother) seemed sexual ("this is certainly not a father-daughter relationship," said the representatives of the wife and daughter).

It was difficult for Ada to accept her mother, who both in her everyday life and in the person of her representative behaved "artificially" in her opinion. Well, she may have had characteristics of a hysterical person, which is often the case with women whose relationship with their father is sexualized. Obviously, Ada could not stop this "harmful relationship" because it is impossible to stop the relationship with the mother. She also rejected potentially successful relationships because there is no substitute for the relationship with the mother.

NEW FAMILIES AND EX-PARTNERS

People have always entered into new relationships and started new families. Although this alone does not violate any orders, many difficulties may arise in such situations. A new relationship and a new family are built on what already existed. Every new partner is the next partner, and the previous ones do not disappear. The new family is connected to the previous family. Therefore, there are no completely new families for those who were in a relationship before or had a child. And yet, we often delude ourselves that we start again, from scratch, really now. Someone who cuts himself off from his previous relationship is deeply involved in it. A man, leaving his woman and child, feels guilty. When he denies the previous relationship, it intensifies. This makes him unable to be fully in the new relationship. The same is true for a woman who pushes away the father of her first child—she also remains tied to him and cannot fully enter into a relationship with a new partner.

And what happens to children born in new relationships? Hellinger notes that if former partners are not respected, these children identity with them. They have various psychological problems because of this. That is why it is important that the second wife, thinking of her husband's first partner, can say, "You are the first, I am the second." So that the man does not try to create everything "from scratch" and agrees that the "old" will always be with him. So that the former partners, whoever they are, are respected and find a place in the memory and heart.

If the relationship ends after many years, and there is no child in it because neither of the partners wanted it, there may be more than just grief at the end. There may also be grief over the lack of a child. When a man and a woman are together, the child always potentially exists. For it is the goal of any such encounter. Nature is not interested in them talking to each other and having a nice time, it is oriented toward procreation, and the unconscious psyche is perfectly aware of this. Therefore, the longer a woman and a man are with each other, even if they do not think about a child, the child starts to be present on the inner level, as a goal of this encounter, which becomes increasingly noticeable to their unconscious. If, however, despite the passage of years, the child is not born, they must say goodbye to its inner image.

A successful relationship is usually hindered by another relationship and another bond. Someone is already related, so they cannot fully get involved in the relationship. It may be someone from not only the family of origin but also the former partner. Melissa could not get pregnant for 5 years with her current partner, 15 years earlier, she had an abortion, then she married the father of the child, but quickly left him. I set her up (in person), her ex-husband, and child. She said she wanted to "get rid of this," "so that it wouldn't exist." She meant the child. The husband was initially angry, he wanted to kick the object representing the child. I said, "You're alike: you don't want to have a child" (the ex-husband lived alone and had no children).

At the end of the constellation, Melissa felt connected to her ex-husband, and they both acknowledged their child. Why could she not start a family? Because she already had one. In the constellation, it became clear, and Melissa felt it. She had previously shut out the fact of her consciousness, and that is why she stayed in a state of limbo. Now she could return to her first family and recognize its importance. I asked her if she wanted to start a new family. She was not ready for that.

Some women got pregnant at an early age and had an abortion. The father of the child may have been a "random boy" who was not interested in either the mother or the child, and quickly vanished. The woman forgot about him and waited for a new, this time "real," relationship. However, it did not come. Why? Because, despite all the unpleasant circumstances, her first relationship was serious, and she did not respect it. Any relationship where there is conception is important and should be treated as a marriage. The next relationship can only be successful if we enter into it with this awareness.

There is a kind of hierarchy between the systems—the new family has some kind of priority over the old one. There is no contradiction here. When a man who already has a family has a child with another woman, then a new family system is created that demands priority over the old one. The man who has the child with the new partner should leave the previous one and get involved with the new one. These are strong words and every man can do as he wishes. However, when a child is born, and thus a new system is formed, a systemic pressure emerges, which somehow pushes him out of one system and attracts to the other. The natural dynamics of such a situation is, therefore, despite all the difficulties involved, to leave the existing family and start the new one. If the man does not commit himself to the next child, this will always have greater consequences than leaving his previous family.

However, all this is not easy at all. Although the hidden dynamics demands that he stay with the new woman and her child, his conscience always holds him to his previous family. The former family remains "first." Therefore, for example, the children of this family remain more important to the man than the new partner. And she must assent to it. Is it all easy? Of course not. That is why we see how many things remain unsettled in patchwork families. New children are often abandoned because the man stays with his former partner. And many men who become involved with new women are only partly with them and with their new families, as the hidden loyalty still keeps them internally with the former families. And the more they cut themselves off from it, do not remember it, or want to start "all over again," the stronger this mechanism is.

For each next relationship is—in a sense—weaker than the previous one. We try not to notice it sometimes, but it is easy to see it in life.

NOTES

1. Quotation translated from German.
2. On the collective level, Hellinger sees this process in the feminist movement. After all, its participants demand "historical justice" for the harm done to many generations of women.

Chapter 5

The Oedipus Complex from a New Perspective

The Oedipus complex is an important concept of psychoanalysis. What is this complex? It is a set of drives, feelings, fears, and desires directed to parents, characteristic of both sexes. It develops because the child directs his or her libidinal desire to the parent of the opposite sex, while the same-sex parent becomes the target of his or her hostile and competitive impulses. This is the basic form of the Oedipus complex, which does not exclude love for the parent of the same sex, and envy or rivalry toward the parent of the opposite sex. As one can see, the Oedipus complex involves ambivalent feelings and both hetero- and homosexual impulses. In addition, the desire to eliminate one parent and own the other is accompanied by fear and guilt as well as a hidden hope that it will not be fulfilled. However, as a psychic remnant of the situation that took place between the mother, father, and child, it affects the lives of adult people, shaping their intimate and professional relationships, ways of interacting with their own children, and often their well-being.

The dynamics that can be described as Oedipal occur in constellations and take the form of admiration, identification, or almost erotic clinging to the parent of the opposite sex, as well as of contempt, rejection, or isolation from the parent of the same sex. Such a situation breaks the orders of love, because, first, the parents are equal in importance, and second, the son is to "stand by his father's side," and the daughter "by her mother's side." As for the erotic aspect of these relationships, while it is a taboo subject in everyday life, and it would not be easy to talk about it, constellations enable an almost tangible contact with Oedipal sexuality. This does not happen in the sphere of the therapist's guesses or conclusions—it is the client, sometimes with the help of a representative, but without any suggestion, who realizes the erotic components of his relationship with the parent, as well as his competitive or rejecting attitude toward the other parent.

Constellations proved, however, that the feelings and situations that psychoanalysis describes as Oedipal have a broad background. It is not just what happens in the child, the parents' attitude is also important, which in turn has transgenerational roots.

Rosalie said her problem was a conflict in her family, between her husband and their son. She said that although she loved "both the men," she loved her son more and stressed that this love was not "unhealthy." The constellation showed that she did not see her son as a son—she saw her first beloved in him. This caused a *quasi*-erotic attitude toward him. This dynamics is frequent—the child often represents the mother's or the father's ex-partner.

Josephine wanted to work on the relationship with her son, who grew apart from her, did not tell her everything, and yet he was "the most important man in her life." The son was 35 years old, and had a wife and three children. Josephine's 90-year-old mother lived in a "private retirement home," and her father had died several decades earlier. The client, speaking about the feud with her brother over the parents' house, made a slip of the tongue twice: "After my mom . . . I mean my father died," "I was supposed to get my mom's part . . . my father's part." Josephine set up a figurine representing her, then I asked her to position the parents too. She set up the mother, but after a while she said that she would "exchange" the mother figurine into her figurine and vice versa. She also added her husband without my suggestions. Later, the son, his wife, and children were brought in, and finally the grandfather and great-grandmothers. It was obvious that it was difficult for the client to take from her mother. The mother was constantly sick, she went to sanatoriums, and the grandmother excused her, saying that she had to understand that her mother was sick. Josephine wanted her figurine to stand with her back to the women in her family.

Then I changed her figurine to a small one—her difficulty approaching the mother and grandmother disappeared. The child wanted to be close. I said that those were her real needs, that she was largely a child, and the client confirmed it. In the further part of the constellation, I again set up the figurine of an adult woman to represent the client, and we worked on her relationship with the son. Finally, the figurines of Josephine and her husband stood opposite their son, his wife, and children. The last sentences of strength uttered on behalf of the son were: "I'm your son," "Here's my wife," "These are our children."

The constellation showed how Josephine's attitude toward her son was determined by her Oedipal relationship with the parents. Josephine wanted to get rid of her mother (slips of the tongue) and take her place (exchange of their figurines). She expressed strong emotions and cried only when she talked about her father's death. She played out her unresolved Oedipus complex in the relationship with her son, who, like her father, became "the most important man" to her. She ignored her husband and did not consider him to be important.

Cynthia never met her father, who was Arab, and left her mother probably when she was pregnant. The first constellation made it possible for her to see and feel that her father felt connected to her, that she was not indifferent to him. During the consultation before the second constellation, she spoke about difficulties in her marriage and the huge hatred for her husband. She also talked about things that could be described as problems with her sense of identity, life goals, work, and having children. She said that she wanted to have sex only sporadically. She also said about the husband's fantasies, which she could not measure up to, but later she added something, "Hmm, maybe I'm alike in this respect."

I stood as her father. Cynthia immediately felt better. I said to her what I felt in that role, "I'm your father. I'm here. I know you're my daughter and I'm your father." It brought Cynthia great relief and joy. She said at one point, "I'm not afraid of it anymore." I asked, "Of what?" Cynthia: "I don't know . . . war . . . " Then I said, "Your father is here, other men and your life are there." However, Cynthia said that she felt uneasy when I mentioned other men. She could not explain it, she just said, "Somehow I can't associate my father with men." I said, "You don't need to associate them." The client sighed and said it was right this way. Then she thought about her husband and felt that now she was looking at him differently, that she could have children with him.

What was the point of this constellation? In my opinion, Cynthia's confusion resulted from a certain fantasy. It boils down to the fact that a woman who has not known her father may be afraid that she may have sexual intercourse with him. Of course, this fantasy is ambivalent—it includes the desire to have sex with her father and the fear of it. An important element here is the unconscious sense of probability of such a situation, perhaps resulting from the existing bond that aims to be revealed. The client said, "I'm not afraid of it anymore." This meant that she was not afraid that she would not recognize her father and that there would be incest. This, however, she could not utter or fully realize. It would have been unnecessary, too traumatic anyway. She slightly forced the association with "the war." When the father became a more real figure, her being a woman became more coherent and the relationship with her husband more possible.

Eloise, a twenty-year-old student, said that her problem was the relationships in the family, intimate relationships with men were even more of a problem, and the issue of sexuality was "a complete disaster." She never had a boyfriend, and when a man accosted her, she felt extremely tense and therefore avoided any conversations and contacts. She had four half-siblings—three sisters and a brother who was the oldest, they were the mother's children, from her first marriage. She said there was one more half-brother who died when he was thirteen. The mother's first husband died from alcohol-related complications. At the second meeting, Eloise said she had had a dream. Someone chased her through a maze-like house, she ran down the stairs, that person had a knife, there were also the siblings and dogs who always showed the chasing one where the chased ones were. She had a suitcase; she wanted to keep it clean. She said that that dream might have been related to her previous therapy—that she "ran away" from certain threads. In the context of the dream, she also said there had been an event "involving her father and a knife." I understood that he could have threatened someone with it or something like that.

I facilitated the constellation using figurines. I asked how her figurine felt; Eloise replied that the figurine was too close to the center (although it stood at the edge). I had the impression that it "was looking at the floor." I said that I would put another figurine in front of her figurine and see "what it would be like." I added the parents and siblings, also the dead brother and the mother's first husband. After a few moves everyone seemed to be looking at the lying person. I placed the figurine of the father next to the dead brother—the client responded saying she had wanted to do it before. They reached peace, turning face to face. The mother could get a little closer and the figurine of the client could stand further away. Eloise said her mother wanted to lie down by her son and husband. I also saw it and put her next to them, with the words, "She can try it, for a moment." The mother seemed to be staring inwardly at the dead son and husband, and Eloise was probably heading toward them instead of her.

When the mother was lying next to her deceased son and his father, the figurines of the client and her father were standing apart from them and from each other. Then I said to Eloise, "When your mother is lying here, only they (I pointed to the figurines of her and the father) can keep their distance, they are not so connected with it. It brings them together. But how can one get closer to the father when there is no mother? It's like trying to replace her. It causes fear. Maybe this is why it's so hard to approach men? Can it be true?" The client replied, "I think so." Then I added, "But the father can be approached, fear is not necessary" (I slowly moved the client figurine and put it closer to the father). In addition to the course of the constellation, I took into account the dreams and associations the client had shared with me (father, knife, gun, suitcase). Showing her the relationship structure and placing the client next to her father was an impulse that made her stop her previous unconscious fantasizing.

Daria was a woman in her thirties, she had two sons, and she was a graduate of three faculties and an owner of an engineering company. Her husband, who was persuaded by her to obtain a secondary education, worked physically. She said her husband attacked her verbally and she wanted to leave him. She expected that this could even improve his contact with the children. Daria's older son had symptoms suggestive of Asperger's syndrome. After a series of moves, the client set up a small figure to represent her son and a large one to represent his father. They stood facing exactly the same direction and with arms stretched in the same way. When I drew her attention to that, she said, "They kind of understand each other without words." I had the impression that they were standing without mutual contact, and yet as if they had something in common. I asked if the husband and son behaved in a similar way.

Client: Yes! He arranges everything nicely, although he doesn't care what he dresses. He has to put everything in order. He has such a great ability to segregate. When he is to bore a hole, he orders his drills and tools.

Therapist (pointing to the figurines of the father and son): They are looking in the direction of the father. This is a longing for the father.

The client said that in fact the husband's relationship with his father is very similar to what the son has with him. At some point of the constellation, all the sons stood close to the figurines of Daria and her father. The client and her father looked like the parents of those children. The husband and real father of the sons stood far behind. I positioned the client in front of her mother. The client said, "I feel kind of jealous that I have good contact with my father too."

The client was strongly attached to her father, his intelligence impressed her, and she chose the same profession. When she talked about how her father raised her, the punishments he used, she cheered up, her eyes began to shine, and her fascination was evident. Her mother was too ordinary for her, gray in her home and female roles, and the daughter basically despised her. I suggested that she bow to the mother, as well as to the earlier women in the family, for the client seemed to despise femininity itself.

C: Yes, I can see it now, she let me educate myself . . .
T: No! She gave birth to you and fed you.
C (Agitated, looking at the mother): Yes.
I set up other women from her family.
C: Indeed, my grandmother had twelve children, she was probably even less appreciated and respected.

I suggested that she say the following words to her father, "I'm just your daughter. I often thought I was your partner. But I'm the daughter." Daria stressed, "A partner has nothing to do with sex." Anyway, it was some kind of partnership and Daria chose a husband who could not measure up to her father and become her partner.

Forty-year-old Charles came for the next constellation, saying that his problem was loans. He constantly took new loans so that his company could function. During the conversation, however, I noticed another problem that seemed more substantive to me and we decided to work on it. Charles "was afraid of people," which was manifested, for example, through his fear when someone entered his store. This is obviously not the best attitude for a salesman. Helped by an assistant, I facilitated the constellation using a static technique—I asked the client to sit on a chair, and invited the assistant to sit on the opposite chair and represent this "what was the problem."

Charles could not look at the representative, who felt confident, a bit amused, and knew that "sooner or later he would look anyway." I sat on a chair next to Charles as "the reason for his fears, for the inability to look," and I myself felt that I was afraid to look, I turned sideways and cowered. Charles calmed down and could now look at the representative. It became clear that I represented some childlike part of Charles, and my assistant—his mother. I told him that it was the mother who was terrifying—just as any mother for a boy—that it was the fear of her femininity. I added a chair next to the mother and sat down as the client's father. Charles was trembling and said that his "legs and balls" were shaking. His father's presence was positive for him, but not really important. I left the role of the father and set up a chair representing him. I positioned it between Charles and his mother, as if separating them, which the mother felt as good—she got tired of her son's attention. Charles calmed down too.

I sat down next to Charles as "something else that also mattered here" and immediately adopted a nonchalant, defiant pose of a "wangler." Charles instantly said that it was him, that he was like that, and that he wished to get rid of "this jelly"—he pointed to himself. We worked on the fact that both those parts were him, that he could not get rid of any of them. We both felt that the difference between us started to disappear. Charles allowed himself to integrate the parts.

Later in the constellation, we worked on Charles's movement toward his mother. I asked him to come closer to the representative of the mother. Charles grabbed the representative by the thighs, bowed his head. For some time I wanted to believe that he was accepting his mother as a mother, but Charles corrected me, saying that he wanted to "take her on his lap" and embrace her "just like a girl." It looked as if the representative had appealed to him, but I knew that we were still in the constellation and that the mother was crucial here. I asked him to turn his chair 180 degrees and I placed a chair opposite, where I sat down the assistant who now represented the "woman," Charles's potential or present partner. What happened was really interesting—Charles said that he lost interest completely and his arousal subsided.

During the session, he felt that his blood pressure was rising, he felt pressure in his head, which he associated with his mother's hypertension. I took it as his identification with her. These symptoms appeared several times and—as indicated by the course of the session—could be considered a defense against his sexual desire for the mother and a sense of her lack as a mother. When he "turned" into the mother, he could not lose her, he also adopted a nonconfrontational attitude toward his father.

Although the process of therapy was progressing, tremors returned, Charles began to feel nausea, "something in his stomach," and a desire to vomit. At first I did not know what it was attributable to, but after a while it became clear that it was still the same thing—the mother and the intermixing of the child's need for the mother, his Oedipal sexuality, and fear of it. I asked Charles to lie down on the mattress. His mother's representative embraced him. This is how we worked on his original bond with the mother. He said then that he thought of the movie *A.I. Artificial Intelligence* that he had watched many times and that kept affecting him. He said that the film unfortunately ended badly, because "the boy stayed with his mother for one night." A moment later, he uttered more or less the same sentence, but this time described the ending of the film as positive. Did he mean that it was "a night with the mother" or that it was "one night"?

The client calmed down not only thanks to the process itself but also thanks to the verbal interpretation, talking about his confusion toward the mother, naming his sexual desires and fears that arose from them. Charles was Oedipally related to his mother, which in turn caused that he did not have a mother as a mother. Or maybe it was rather the interruption of the early bond that made him cling to his mother Oedipally? Whatever it was, both processes strengthened each other. The moment when the mother clearly said to her son that he was a child and she was with his father was an important part of the constellation. What brought relief to the client was also the possibility to sit in front of his father and hear his words: "You can be like me." These words do not push a son to take the place of his father, on the contrary—they aid in masculine identification with him and going his own way. Charles also understood the meaning of loans in his life—he wanted to "vomit" them, and yet he kept taking them. During this session, there was a moment when he spontaneously visualized himself as a bamboo tree "empty inside." In fact, he wanted to take from the mother, but was unable to.

Bianca's constellation concerned her son, who began to act impulsively, knocked objects, hit her, and said that she did not understand what he was going through.

T: How did you feel about your son then?

C: I was definitely angry . . . I felt—sorry, I will say it straight—like a cunt. I felt like a woman who was treated undeservedly this way.

Bianca felt like a "cunt" and "woman," not like a mother who did not deserve her son's attitude. In the constellation, Bianca stood in person, and on the floor we put two sheets of paper—marked as "Mark" (her son) and the "father" (her son's father). When the client stood in front of me (I represented her son), she began to smile and was excited. The son looked her in the eye. When I asked her to imagine that she stood face to face with her husband and with her side to the son, she found herself uncomfortable about Mark's presence. At this point, as the son, I felt what I could call "moderate madness," as if I was lost and confused. Something strange was happening to me, I could not tell if it was something terrifying or exciting, avoided or expected. Ultimately, however, that union of the parents was desirable and liberating. At some point, Bianca said that her son used to snuggle up to her all the time. It annoyed her and she told him that she would not be his wife. It was supposed to show him the real situation. However, I felt differently and asked her to describe the context of that situation. She said she had talked with the sons about darning. Mark said that now she darned for him, and then his wife would do it. It was clear that the son was trying to separate the future wife from the mother, and it was the client who linked them.

When the client told the story "about the wife," I (still representing the son) moved away quite abruptly—the son did not want that type of projection. During the constellation, the client found her feelings for her son as erotic, as one could have for a partner. She also wondered why the son was so aggressive. The further course of the constellation lent credence to the hypothesis that he felt lonely, abandoned by his father, and used by the mother.

Paul wanted to work on the relationship with his wife, who had suffered from depressive states for a long time. I saw some kind of fear in his attitude and the way he talked about his wife. I was strongly convinced that his mother was important here. After a moment of silence, I asked if there was anything else that could be relevant too. Paul said he was recalling a memory of peeping at his mother through the ventilation grille in the bathroom door. I asked if he liked it, to let him express his excitement. Paul confirmed.

I set up Paul's representative and his mother's representative. His representative recounted embarrassment mixed with excitement. He did not look his mother in the face and turned his side to her. I offered the mother the sentence: "You're just a boy."

What did I aim at? At the restoration of the interrupted relationship with the parent by indicating that "nothing serious had happened." Paul's representative became more confident and finally could look at his mother. I positioned the representatives of Paul's father and wife, and asked the client himself to stand and replace his representative. The client felt that he would like to lie down on the floor and look under the skirt of the mother's representative. He showed no interest in his wife. I said, "Yes, the fascination with the mother is the strongest." And then, humorously, pointing to his father standing next to the mother, "He's done 'worse' things with her." Finally, I asked the parents to turn to their son and I said, "That one is just a dream."

Paul turned to his wife's representative and said that he only now noticed her and could look at her.

Chapter 6

Systemic Aspects of Gender Identity

In this chapter, I would like to address the issue of male and female gender identity. There is no doubt that there are differences in the extent and manner in which people identify with a given gender. The experience of being a woman or being a man is not the same for everyone. Some people have no problems with their own gender, for others the subject remains questionable. Some feel good in their male or female body, others feel bad. There are people who do not mind their undefined or conflicted attitude to their own sex, but there are many who suffer because of it. These people would like to be more "female" or "male." Thanks to therapeutic work, such as constellations, we can see that this or that attitude to gender is not a coincidence, nor does it need to be biologically conditioned. It more often results from a certain psychological history.

The subject of gender identity covers a whole spectrum of cases. Perhaps the most extreme attitudes to the gender issue are displayed in transsexual people, who, despite having anatomical features peculiar to the given gender, identify with the opposite one. There are also those who cannot assign themselves to any category within the binary gender classification—neither as a woman nor as a man.[1]

On the other hand, there may be more subtle gender-related problems. One can have a husband or wife with this problem and never notice it, and even more—the person affected by the problem may also be unaware of it. This hidden problem does not have to manifest itself directly—in the form of identification with the opposite sex or a consciously experienced feeling of uncertainty about one's gender role. It can manifest itself in the form of various difficulties in relationships, in assuming the role of a parent, and even in difficulty finding one's place at work (of course, all these issues can also be conditioned by completely different causes). In a constellation, however, we can discover that the above problems concern precisely the broadly understood issue of "femininity" and "masculinity." It is not a question of any abstractions, but the attitude to one's own gender, resulting, for example, from a woman's rejection of her mother and female line, or a man's rejection of his father.

It is possible to speak of male or female identification because the existence of two sexes is a fact, which is related to the process of reproduction, which is sexual. This biological fact entails complex psychological dynamics. Thanks to constellations, we realize that male and female roles have deep roots, even if they are associated with cultural stereotypes (to which some would like to reduce all factors that shape the differences between women and men). This is because the division into women and men has lasted for thousands of years. During this time, billions of people recorded these patterns in the morphic field. Therefore, even if someone has problems with gender identification or would like to avoid any identification, they are faced with a "woman" and "man" as archetypes and behavioral attractors.

Let us pay attention to one characteristic circumstance: transsexual people are capable of making great sacrifices to become similar to the gender they identify with (we cannot speak of real "sex change" here, as it is sometimes called). They are willing to sacrifice erectile and erogenous organs, such as the penis and clitoris, they agree to remain infertile, to take artificial hormones for most of their lives. The strength of their conviction that they "really" are of another gender is also amazing. One mother wrote that her transsexual son (M/F transsexualism) "loved to be a girl, probably the most of all girls in the world."

Isn't there anything amazing about it? How can one love so much? Or rather: who does one love this way? Being mindful of the principles of systemic constellations, we know that such great love, going beyond self-care, is addressed to people from the family system. Especially those whose fate one is entangled in.

In some cases, only partial transformation is desired, as is the case with transvestism. The basic mechanism, however, is similar and consists in identification with some woman from the system. This is what one man said about his youth, now dressed as a woman, but having sexual relations with a woman, "Even then, I had a sense of super-split personality, I wanted to be half-and-half [half-woman, half-man], but I couldn't. I dreamed of stopping it, and I thought maybe a doctor would help me, that there is a cure for it" (Słodkowski 2014). When he assumed the appearance of a woman, he felt much better mentally: "I'm not so unstable internally and I don't have those mood swings, so others also feel better with me. I lifted a great weight off myself" (Słodkowski 2014). When the man was a child, he behaved like a typical boy, he also had boyish interests (toy soldiers, football). Interestingly, he also said, "But sometimes I dress like a man, go out and feel great relief that nobody pays attention to me" (Słodkowski 2014).[2]

In similar cases, the parents' attitude may play a role here. It happens that a man says that his parents "wanted a girl" and a woman—that her parents "wanted a boy." These people grow up with the feeling that their deep, gender-related self is rejected. What could be the reason that the mother does not accept the boy and wants a girl, or vice versa? Constellations show that the reason could be the siblings who died before. It happens that the mother cannot accept her child's death, and her way to reduce pain is the fantasy that the child will be born again. However, when a child of a different sex is born, the mother may feel comfortless. Then she (more or less consciously) rejects the sex of her child. As a result, the child, desiring the mother's love, hides and suppresses the fullness of manifestations of his sex. However, what generally pushes toward identification with the gender other than the biological one is the entanglement with a person from the family—a woman in case of a boy and a man in case of a girl.

At the age of 18, Robert married a girl with whom he had a daughter. When we talked, he was in his thirties and he told me that he had been immature all those years, that he did not fully accept his relationship. He confessed that he fantasized about killing his wife and daughter, which would give him freedom. Recently, he told his wife he had cheated her a few times with prostitutes. He said that his wife was valuable to him, that their relationship strengthened, and that he would like to become more mature and ready to assume his male role. Robert was aware of many hidden aspects of his personality, for example, his phallic-narcissistic traits. He said that he had thought of his penis as a separate entity for a long time, as a better version of himself, seeing his power in it. On the other hand, he was always a "good boy," raised by strong women, his mother and grandmother, and he described his father as rather subordinate. He also said that he himself was still trying to be "well-behaved." I responded that when we had talked on the phone, he had had a very pleasing way of expressing himself. He answered that he was often taken for a woman by his interlocutors (his work involved telephone conversations). It was unusual because the timbre of his voice was by no means high, but fully masculine.

I facilitated an individual constellation. I intuitively chose the element that I described as "the person who matters here." I stood in front of the client, looking in his eyes. I said to him, "I'm a woman." Later, I felt someone else was also important there. I left the role of the "woman" and took this new position. I felt that it was a man. There was something very aggressive and traumatic in his relationship with that woman, probably also sexual. It seemed to be a case of the perpetrator and the victim. Robert identified with both the perpetrator and the victim, with the woman and the man. These identifications were the reason for his conflict between the murderous fantasies and courtesy, male phallicism and female subordination.

The point was to stick to his "ordinary" male role. When I stood in the place of the man, I said to the client, "I'm a man too." These words appeared spontaneously, but paradoxically freed the client from equating masculinity with extreme aggression, as if it had been said: "We are men, but we can be different."

A boy needs male energy flowing from the male line of his family. Its direct and most important transmitter is his father. When the transmission from the father to the son is blocked, when the son cannot "stand by his father," his development as a man, and even as an internally coherent and strong person, is at risk. This is demonstrated by the following constellation.

Rita had no respect for her husband, which she openly admitted. She also did not respect him as their daughter's father. In turn, the daughter pushed away the father of her children, her son and daughter. She did not value him, she considered him weak, and her representative was indifferent to him. What was happening to the son of Rita's daughter in this situation? The four-year-old boy experienced a great inner anxiety, which was observable by the representative of the child. The age of the son, who was in the Oedipal period, could also play a role. Unable to count on the support of his father's energy and his function to separate him from the mother, the boy was exposed to the feeling of terror associated with the all-pervading mother.

In the Oedipus period, the boy obviously "desires to possess his mother and eliminate the father," but at the same time, he is very afraid of this and prefers not to. In this situation, the child's way out can be a more complete identification with the mother, a kind of psychic surrender to her. This identification means that he is no longer face-to-face with his mother, so she ceases to be a sexual object. He is now "on the same side of the fence." After the constellation, when I shared these observations with the group, a person from Rita's family present in the room said that this boy had his nails painted and that he used the grammatical feminine form.[3]

Gender identity and sexual orientation are different, but mutually interpenetrating areas. Therefore, in the context of identification with the opposite gender, we can also talk about homosexuality. Hellinger distinguishes two main types of homosexuality: caused by identification with someone of the opposite sex or with a marginalized and excluded person (because being homosexual, at least until modern times, translated into being an outsider). Basically, he does not distinguish homosexuality (at least of the first type) from gender identity problems. Indeed, in all such cases I know, in constellations, we discover unconscious identifications with the opposite sex. However, constellations do not make it possible to determine why a given person is bisexual, another one is homosexual, why someone becomes transsexual and wants a sex reassignment surgery, and why someone else only experiences difficulties as a man or woman, adopting certain features characteristic of the opposite gender. There seem to be other reasons behind this variety. This awareness, along with general respect for clients as free people, protects against hasty attempts to change one's sexual preferences.

Martin was a twenty-year-old man. He did not accept his homosexuality. He said that he would like to enter into a relationship with a woman, that he believed only in this kind of relationship; however, women did not excite him at all. On the other hand, after he had sex with men, he did not feel well, he wanted the partner to disappear as soon as possible. Sometimes he told himself this was the last time, but after some time the desire for sex returned, and the situation recreated in his imagination became exciting. Martin had a sister two years older, whom he described as "anti-relational," emphasizing that he had a completely different view on this—he wanted a relationship, but he could not imagine it with a man. He saw "how it looked," that "those relationships were generally superficial or failed at all." He always had a stronger relationship with his mother than with his father. The parents often argued. He never had good contact with his peers—he did not play football, did not do sports, he rather stayed at home—but he was impressed by boldness and independence of many classmates. He was excited when no one bothered on class trips to which bed they lay, so he slept in the beds of his mates.

I asked Martin to use figurines to set up himself and his sister. He put his sister by himself, he had a feeling that they wanted to take each other's hands, so he brought the figurines closer. I asked him to add the parents. Martin put his father by his sister and the mother by himself. The figurines of the sister, client, and mother stood in one line and looked straight ahead. The father was positioned in a way that he looked behind their backs. I asked Martin how the family members felt. "No one feels good here," he replied. The relations were static, as if nullifying any movement. I set up the mother in front of the father. Martin and his sister felt anxious, which was interesting for him. In the further course of the constellation, I intuitively positioned the father's father behind the father. It changed the mother's feelings, she moved away a bit. Martin said that his mother never liked the grandfather, she always had a grudge against him, but the grandfather did not dispute, he was a calm man. Martin placed his mother by him again. I added the mother's father. The client said, pointing to the figurines, "Like here, as if with disgust, but there's a connection." He meant the mother standing with her father and his father standing with his sister and holding her hand. At this point, a thought came to my mind about possible sexual abuse caused by the grandfather ("disgust," "connection").

During the constellation Martin spontaneously pointed out his sister's ambivalent attitude toward the father several times: her desire to be close and antipathy. The mother's mother and mother's sister and brother were also set up. Martin made a string of the figurines holding one another's hands. Only the mother's brother, an alcoholic, stood outside that row. At that moment, Martin had the sister on one side, the mother on the other, and further also the mother's mother and mother's sister. He was standing in the row of women.

Eventually, the constellation could come to the moment when Martin's parents stood behind him and his sister, the mother's siblings more to the side, the parents' parents even more to the back, which expressed a systemic order. I set up a woman figurine in front of Martin. It was his potential partner, a person he wanted a relationship with. Then I also positioned a man, the sister's potential partner. The following sequence of feelings and associations of the client was extensive, which is why I describe them in brief. When the potential partner appeared, Martin's sister wanted to hold his hand tighter. His parents looked at him and his partner approvingly. Also, the father's father looked as if he wanted to come closer and support this situation. The sister's potential partner approached and moved away in response to her rejection. Martin remembered that his sister had once said, "How can you love a stranger? You can love someone you have known since childhood, someone close to you." I asked, "Would the following words 'I'm scared' be appropriate for your sister?." "Oh, yes, very," said Martin.

It was evident that the sister was afraid of getting out of the chain of the figurines holding one another, and in particular of her close relationship with the brother. There was an interesting connection here, as if he identified with the sister by taking over her fears. Martin shared her fear, that is, the fear of leaving their relationship, of a romantic relationship, of a man, of leaving the family. Martin also had his own fear—of being left alone, without the sister. During the sequence with potential partners, he was interested in both the woman and man, but when his sister could get closer to the man, Martin lost interest in him, and at the same time, his interest in the woman increased. The sister was interested in Martin's woman only as a possible rival.

As it can be seen, Martin identified with women and took over their attitudes. His relationship with the sister was particularly strong and could have led to Martin's ego-dystonic (unaccepted) homosexuality. In the family system, the hierarchical relationship was replaced by a "chain." Both the succession of generations and entering into new relationships as a recipe for loneliness were negated.

Homosexuality could be a way to stick to the family system. The erotic relationship with the sister, fear of losing her, her jealousy, and anger could also lead to avoiding relationships with women. Added to this was the desire to relieve her by being always close. Also, perhaps the client "brought" men into his sister's life to tame her fear (as if he said, "Look, men are not so bad"). Martin's homosexuality would be "homosexuality for the sister."

Collin was a homosexual man in his twenties, and he was anorexically thin. His problem—as he presented it—was that "he absorbed everything into himself" and that it manifested in his body, which was tense, as well as in his emotions, because anger accumulated in him and sometimes he exploded without any apparent reason. He said that he eventually "got up in the morning and puked" (literally). He had a brother, a few years older than him. The brother—as it was presented in the family—was "worse," Collin was better because he was "polite," because he "learned." Collin said he did not have good contact with his father, but he had very good contact with the mother, with whom he talked on the phone every day. They confided in each other, although usually the mother did it.

Collin chose a woman to represent him. In the constellation, at first, his mother did not look at him, but somewhere into the distance. I positioned "what the mother was looking at." Later in the constellation, I added the father and brother. The mother embraced "what she was looking at." Collin said that he did not know if it was relevant, that it probably was not, but the mother had a twin sister. It was the most important dynamics—the mother's relationship with her twin sister, or more precisely, the mother's need to have someone very close. The constellation showed that the mother desired someone like her to be next to her, like the second part of herself. Her representative said to the sister, "I thought we would always be together." The mother transferred this need to her son, who became a part of herself in a way. In the constellation, one could observe a kind of rivalry between Collin and the mother's sister. That is why it was extremely difficult for Collin to utter the key sentence of strength: "I have nothing to do with it" in relation to his mother's relationship with her sister. He had slightly less difficulty saying the sentence: "You're my mother, I accept you as a mother. I'm just a child." The constellation also showed a problem in the relationship with the father and a peculiar division into men and women. On one side stood Collin's father and brother, on the other—his mother and sister. Collin stood in the middle—he connected what is male and female.

In the constellation, we see several elements that can be associated with homosexual orientation. It was probably determined in many ways, but the love for the mother seemed to be the most important thing here. Being his mother's confidant, and thus also violating the hierarchy, made Collin's existence unique ("better"). He preserved this uniqueness in the form of sexual distinctness (especially in relation to his heterosexual brother). Perhaps he felt that he had to be special to keep the love of his mother, who was so strongly attached to her sister. In addition, he held the family together by combining what was male and female. The boy "did not need" a father, but his unconscious and body signaled that what his mother "poured into him" was not good food—he was losing her as a mother, and "swallowed" her unfulfilled desires that were indigestible in the long run. Hence thinness, vomiting, accumulated anger.

During a constellation training course, Lucia said she had an arthritis problem in her hands. She also said there was some unresolved issue between her father and mother. I asked someone from the group to represent Lucia. The representative said that she felt as if she was climbing a rope, higher and higher, and that she could not afford to be at the bottom. She also made the corresponding gesture with her hands, as if she was grabbing the rope. Then Lucia added that as a 10- to 12-year-old child she trained in gymnastics and one of the exercises was climbing high up the rope with a load. The representative also had a vision of the podium, to which Lucia said that she had been the hope of the club, but the jitters had blocked her in the critical competition.

The trainee, who facilitated this constellation under my supervision, added "what was at the bottom," and then also "what prevented her from letting go of the rope." These representatives had associations regarding the negation of femininity—"One needs to be a boy," "One needs to manage." Lucia actually had a masculine way of being and dressed this way, in addition, she said that her father wanted to have a son. So we added "femininity" and the "father." The father tried to cover Lucia's representative's socks with a shawl because they were colorful and feminine. The representative of "what was at the bottom" felt stiffening and unpleasant sensations around the shoulder girdle. Lucia replied that her health problems were concentrated in this area (except for the hand problems). Whereas the representative of "what prevented her from letting go of the rope" became an accuser of the father's actions, she felt that she had to make him aware of the consequences of how he had influenced his daughter (of course, I still mean the feelings from the role and not the conscious attitude of the given trainee).

Finally, we brought in a representative of "the reason why the father behaved this way." The "reason" stood upright with its legs joined together, swinging to the sides. Its representative said she felt like a buoy in the water. Earlier, one of the representatives had said that she had felt as if she had been under the water. Then Lucia said that her father had been born and lived by a large lake, where many people drowned. The constellation got more and more dramatic. The representative of "what was at the bottom" already clearly felt that she was representing some person, most probably a girl. She had a vague impression that someone had contributed to her death, or at least could not save her. The representatives began to see the shawl, which was spontaneously used in the constellation, as a rope. The representative of the drowning girl wanted to get to the surface.

When these matters began to come to light, the representative's accusing attitude toward the father changed, Lucia's representative also started to change it. An explanation began to emerge that the father (perhaps subconsciously) was afraid that as a girl she would not manage, that she needed to be strong like a boy. In this constellation, Lucia felt a strong connection with—probably—the drowned girl and her fate.

We could actually end the work at this stage, but we have also brought in a representative of Lucia's mother. This started a new thread. The mother began to walk around vigorously. After a while, the mother's representative asked if Lucia's mother had a younger brother, because her brother came to her mind. Lucia confirmed. We brought in a representative of the brother. The representative of the mother felt an erotic and loving fascination, but the brother tried to retreat. In this moment, Lucia's brother came to the representatives' minds. Lucia said that she indeed had a brother. We brought him in the constellation.

Eventually, it became almost certain that there was another dynamics leading to the masculinization of the daughter—the mother was afraid that an erotic fascination could also be born between her daughter and son. This assumption was also supported by Lucia's words that sex in her house was "more than a taboo" and that the mother was not even able to say "butt."

As can be seen, the development of our attitude to gender is a very complex and multiway process. And yet we have no reason to believe that the aforementioned dynamics and processes are the only ones in this respect.

NOTES

1. These classification ambiguities lead to attempts to create the so-called third gender or to negate the meaning of gender in general. To somehow define the variety of sense of identity and social phenomena, terms such as gender nonconforming, agender, transgender, genderqueer, gender-fluid, and so forth, are used. It seems that exploring what gender and the difference between genders actually are is a borderline situation of our cognition—for everyone considers gender from the "inside" of their own gender or their problems with gender, unable to objectively grasp the subject.
2. Quotations translated from Polish.
3. In Polish, parts of speech, for example, verbs, have different endings depending on whether the subject in a sentence is a woman or a man.

Chapter 7

Mental and Behavioral Disorders

SYMPTOMS FROM A SYSTEMIC PERSPECTIVE

Certain psychopathological symptoms accompany many disorders. These include anxiety, depression, and various inhibitions in work and personal life. We can consider anxiety as a signal that from the depths of the psyche lets us know that something is wrong. Usually, anxiety persists for years, and it is difficult to deal with it both with the help of pharmacotherapy (anxiolytics are among the most addictive drugs) and psychotherapy. Constellations bring a real breakthrough here because they make it possible to eliminate anxiety or radically reduce it in just one session. When anxiety is taken over from the family system, leaving "what is not mine" is enough for it to subside. Twenty-year-old Cornelia's anxieties came primarily from taking over the anxieties of her mother and grandmother. When she realized this and took the position of a child who could not carry those things, the anxieties immediately ended.

Anxiety, whose causes lie primarily in the subject's personal history may have its source in the prenatal and perinatal periods. In this case, years of psychotherapy, meditation, and relaxation may not be effective. It is only when you experience your own birth again, in its systemic context, that you get out of the recurring anxiety states. Interestingly, this fact is in line with the concept of anxiety of Sigmund Freud, who considered birth to be the prototype situation of anxiety. He also believed—despite later changes and the complexity of his theory—that the unsatisfied libido transforms directly into anxiety, which occurs in anxiety neurosis and children's phobias. And in Freud's concept, the libido is not just the sex drive, but the entirety of "love energy," and it is also associated with the child's need for contact with his mother. Here is what he writes about children suffering from phobia, afraid of strangers:

> Loneliness as well as a strange face arouse the child's longing for his familiar mother; he is unable to control his libidinal excitation, he cannot hold it in suspense but changes it into anxiety. (Freud 1990, 103)

So it is the longing for the mother that causes some anxieties. This accords with our observations, and we understand this longing primarily as a consequence of the disruption of the original bond by external events. The interrupted movement toward the mother, especially if it occurred in the perinatal period, is a deep, unconscious longing for the mother. Then the libido, unsatisfied in contact with the mother, may transform into anxiety. From the point of view of systemic constellations, the unsatisfied libido would be an unsatisfied need to take from the mother with love. In this perspective, it has the dimension of giving and taking—taking what the mother gives and giving gratitude for it. Re-experiencing the way to the mother (in a constellation) redirects the libido to the right object that is the mother, at the same time making it possible to take the position of a child and express gratitude. Then anxiety disappears.

Depressive states are the most common, next to anxiety, psychopathological symptoms. They can vary in severity, ranging from a temporary lack of joy in life to severe depression lasting for years. Leaving the most severe cases aside, depression can be considered a symptom associated with various events and dynamics. Depression may result from the rejection of a parent, the death of an older sibling, or its causes may be transgenerational. Exclusion, secrets, not accepting responsibility, and the like lead to a kind of chaos in the system, which can result in depression of someone completely unaware of these events. It seems that here there may be a phenomenon of gradual accumulation and transformation of psychological material. The process may begin with the grandmother's loss and incomplete mourning; while, however, the grandmother experienced the real thing, that is, the loss, her son experiences an irrational tension related to his mother's mental state, and her grandson experiences depression. In this case, depression has a three-generational structure.

Susceptibility to depressive states, apathy and lack of motivation is also associated with not accepting one of the parents. Hellinger emphasizes that with the acceptance of an excluded or disrespected parent, the basic mood level increases immediately. I remember a training workshop attended by several dozen participants. Although we had done various exercises before, after the exercise that concerned accepting the father there was loud and joyful laughter in all corners of the room. In this way a feeling of relief and regained energy appeared.

We can also see depressiveness as the effect of not taking strength from the entire family, turning away from the ancestors. This is not uncommon in situations where there were many problems and dramas in the family, such as suicides, alcoholism, social degradation, arguments, and animosities. In such cases, the individual "does not want to have anything to do with his family." To a certain extent, he saves his emotional life, but always at a high price. This price is cutting oneself off from the strength that is also present in his family. The only constructive way out, that is, combining the act of leaving the burden with accepting the ancestors, is possible through constellations.

Inhibitions are a common psychopathological symptom. They may concern contacts with people in general or contacts with the opposite sex, or difficulties in carrying out paid or creative work. The background of these states may vary, but a systemic constellation is often a landmark here. Inhibitions may result from being entangled in the fate of a deceased or excluded person. This unconscious bond results in a lack of energy and unwillingness to commit oneself to other relationships and activities.

Despite her great artistic talent, Angelica could not follow her passion, which was painting. She wanted to paint, but she could not start doing it. The longer she told me about her inhibition, the more it became clear that painting could represent a person. Painting was something she often thought about, which was basically within reach yet impossible to do. It was like a person one is attached to, but does not come close to, keeps away from. However, one never forgets about this person. We did not use constellations in our work, but when I told Angelica about my hypothesis, she replied, "Yes, when I'm about to paint, ideas about parting come to my mind." I suggested that she separate painting from the unknown person. Painting is just painting; the bond is with someone else. After this session, she finished a painting that had been unfinished for a few years.

Juliana felt that something blocked her, prevented her from developing, and from living the life she wanted to live. As a representative of this blockade, I lay down on the ground. I was someone dead. Then I put an object as a representation of this person, left the role and represented Juliana's mother and then her grandmother, who seemed important based on what the client said already during the initial interview. Both Juliana's mother and grandmother reacted dramatically to the deceased. Juliana said, "There is life here, with this person." She felt that something was opening up within her and reviving. How is this possible? The deceased person was someone excluded, he evoked sadness and fear. Like a deceased child, whom one does not want to remember. Juliana's mother probably did not come into contact with him personally, but she experienced, in her own way, the fears of her mother, who might have known who it was. Then there was Juliana, who reacted to this transgenerational trauma with an internal blockade of vitality (she told me that in her childhood, when she watched films like *The Adventures of Robin Hood*, she always thought: "There was life there, real life"). Now that she took the departed person into her heart, everything turned out to be not so terrible and her vital forces could finally come.

Constant failures are another common type of problem. These can concern relationships, professional, and financial matters. They are sometimes caused by an unconscious attempt to atone for somebody else's or one's own fault or identification with someone whose lot was hard. The reasons can also be guilt for not accepting one of the parents and an unconscious need for self-punishment.

SELECTED DISORDERS—EXAMPLE CASE STUDIES

Anorexia

Isabel was a 20-year-old girl with anorexia. She could not show affection from an early age, she had no deep relationships with her peers or partner, and she said food was a substitute for deeper relationships for her. Isabel maintained that she was similar to her father, although she had poor contact with him. Her paternal grandfather was an alcoholic, and her grandmother was said to have slept in the same bed with Isabel's father for a long time and spoiled him. She left with her third husband when the son was not of legal age yet.

Representative of Isabel (I): I want to move away from my mother, I'm scared.
Representative of Isabel's mother (M): I feel blocked.
I: It doesn't get through to me, it's new. I see dad as a boy, a weak boy.
M: I'd like to hold her.
I: I feel like I'm dying, my heart is ripping apart. As if I had a son (the father tries to stand arm in arm with the daughter).
M: I feel strong, I know I can help her, but she's running away.
I: But I don't feel I need to stand by my mother. And dad is annoying me. I wish my dad was strong.
(The mother and daughter are laughing.)
M: She's very strong, but she has so much love for this gink (laughter). (A sentence of strength:) "I respect your love for your father. But this is your safe place at the moment. I am big, even though you're strong."

This sequence of the constellation shows the issue of a "weak and withdrawn" father, already observed by traditional therapists and psychologists studying the families of anorexic women. Hellinger also emphasizes that anorexia involves the daughter's solidarity with her father, whom the anorexic wants to stop in his movement, which she sees as a movement toward death or leaving the family. Here is the further part of this constellation.

M: I see my daughter curled up, small, sad. I'm also scared now.
(The therapist positions the mother in front of Isabel and asks Isabel to look at both her parents. At the same time, the mother receives "support"—a representative standing behind her.)
M: I'm tied up in knots.
Therapist: Turn around.
M: As if I saw something new (looking at the representative behind her). I felt such fear; I got so tiny (the indications are that the support is the mother's mother).
The therapist speaking to the mother: Maybe it was you who was such a "small abandoned child." Take a step forward (toward your own mother).
M: I'm so scared, terribly!
T: Can you touch each other carefully?
M: The armor that was on me, that apparent strength, is broken now.
(At the end of the constellation, the parents are standing side by side, behind the client's father—his father, behind the mother—her mother. The representative of Isabel is standing in front of them.)
I: Now I feel I can join them. I just don't know—mom or dad? (She's approaching the father.) Now he's a pillar, it's safe.

Finally, the client herself entered the constellation, she felt "safe and blissful."

The constellation showed that it was difficult not only for the father to take masculine strength from his own father but also the mother was in some respects a "small child" and directed her needs to her daughter. The daughter did not get the support she needed from her parents, because they themselves were cut off from their parents and did not take strength from them.

In classic family psychotherapy, it was observed that anorexia is a kind of intervention directed toward the parent couple. Through her illness, the anorexic integrates the family and creates a common task for the parents. Constellations confirm this general picture, and they make it more detailed and deepened.

During another constellation of an anorexic girl, Emily, I set up a representative of her father in front of her mother. It was difficult for the mother to recognize her partner as the father of their daughter. She took the attitude that I refer to as "parthenogenesis syndrome." She did not fully accept the thought that the child was a fruit of a woman and a man. She did not want to think of her daughter as a child of them both. There was no gratitude to the other parent for having this child. When the women stood opposite each other, the mother was not able to admit the simple fact that Emily had a father. It was obvious that the daughter suffered because of this. The mother repeated, apparently rationally, "First he has to change his behavior toward me and my daughter," which in this situation was just to mask her basic difficulty. Eventually, I suggested the mother say the simplest words: "He fertilized me. You were born of it." It was only after these sentences that the daughter felt relieved.

Anorexia has also other dimensions. In this disease, concentration on the abdomen is very common—it is supposed to be absolutely flat. The smallest meal can make the abdomen grow, so many anorexics provoke vomiting. When they eat something, they feel—as they say—remorse. Based on observations, I hypothesize that the dynamics associated with some form of entanglement in the fate of an (probably unborn) child and his mother may play a part in the picture of anorexia. There would be a peculiar kind of conflict here—the anorexic identifies with the pregnant woman and the fetus, and at the same time rejects this identification, defends herself against it (flat stomach).

During one exercise, when I represented "remorse," which very quickly turned out to be rather a person, probably a child, the aforementioned Emily almost heard a voice in the head: "Don't give in!," which I understand just as an expression of the said defense. At the same time, after this session, she felt better and ate without vomiting for the first time in more than a year. Interestingly enough, she had long dreamed of traveling to Africa to help local children.

The matter of anorexia may be even more complex. Magdalene was less than fifty years old, and the problem she came with was morbid jealousy that prevented her from being in a relationship with any man. From the age of sixteen, she had suffered from anorexia, then bulimia, she had stopped vomiting only three years before the session, but she still controlled eating, and when she ate something, she felt discomfort in the abdominal area. She had a daughter, who had moved away from her two years earlier. We brought up the issue of her sexuality: she masturbated since preschool, later, despite many sexual contacts, she did not get satisfaction, had only a few orgasms. She said she was constantly cold, she was trembling now, and she did not know why. In addition, she felt a painful pressure on her stomach, and later in the conversation, there was also pain in the neck. Magdalene said she was constantly looking critically at herself, at her body.

I asked her to stand up and asked which part of her body she felt most. She said about the pain in the neck and the shoulders. I took a piece of paper and laid it on the floor as "something/someone associated with that pain." I stood on the sheet and immediately approached Magdalene, I looked her in the eye, also at her hands, a little at the body. The client did not know who it might be, but I supposed it was her mother. The person I represented was trying to ask Magdalene, "What's the problem?" as if her expectations surprised her.

I asked what her birth was like. She was born blue, with the umbilical cord around. When she told me about it, the pain in the neck and in the area of the stomach increased, the client doubled up. She said something was strangling her, she started to feel nausea, and she talked about phlegm. Whoever I was, I came near, grabbed Magdalene by the neck with one hand, and I pressed her belly with the other. The client wanted the pressure to be even stronger. It was clearly related to the memory of her birth. After some time, Magdalene calmed down, and I left the role.

Magdalene said that she did not like her body because she was "meant to be a boy," and that she probably disappointed her parents in this regard. I told her that this was "nonsense," that from the point of view of birth—that is, that she existed—all those words of the parents did not matter. There must have been something stronger that kept her in this attitude. I continued the constellation. I stood as Magdalene's mother. I had the same move as before—I walked closer to the daughter. As the mother, I turned Magdalene toward the window and pushed her gently saying that the mother would wish this for her (i.e., that she would go into her life, which is often represented by the view outside the window during the constellations I facilitate). But Magdalene could not do it. She said that half of her was somewhere else, and a moment later added, "I'd like to go back there"—pointing at the mother's belly.

I left the role of the mother, and behind the sheet representing the mother I put another one, saying that it represented "something earlier that matters here." As I stood on that piece of paper, I began to look around the consulting room, touching the shelves. I acted like someone who had just regained eyesight and examined their surroundings. I told the client that it was someone who was not meant to live and asked if there was a child who had died. Magdalene said that in the mother's family there was not, but her father's twin brother had died just after the birth. So it was probably him. As I walked around the room and touched the shelves, the client was scared, she had a feeling that that person wanted to "take her with him." I asked the client to utter certain sentences of strength. She calmed down when she could say, "You have a place in my heart, you live there." After those words, I also became calmer as the representative.

And yet Magdalene still could not fully leave her father's brother. She felt some connection in the body. I asked her if she wanted to get closer. She confirmed. When she approached, I grabbed her hand, then the other, following an impulse, I pulled her closer. She said that there was something sexual about it, that it was horrible, that he was some satiric man. There was indeed something sexual in this, but as the person I represented, I had no bad intentions toward her. There was even an element of tenderness. When I pulled the client closer, she said, "That's my father, that's my father." I asked if there had been anything sexual in her father's behavior. She denied. As I found out, however, this situation was related to the feelings Magdalene had since she had begun to mature—"she was disgusted by men's sexual desire" when they looked at her, and she tried to dress so as to cover as much as possible.

Later in the constellation, I separated the father and his brother. I stood as the father and his brother was represented by an item laid on the floor. The father was moving in a "flustered" manner, just like the brother. He was identified with him. When I finally stood more calmly beside the deceased brother, the client said, "Now I know! I wanted to leave instead of him, of my father." At the end of the constellation, the father said to his daughter that she was free, that he would stay by his brother.

How can we understand all this? Both me and the client realized that the father needed a "body" with which he wanted to merge with. It was not about sexuality and the daughter but about the brother. However, she could perceive it as sexuality and hence the disgust. The father, until he found his way to the twin brother, was not able to find peace. This constellation confirms Hellinger's thesis that the anorexic follows her father. We can see, however, that this movement can be interwoven with complex psychodynamics. In this case, the psychodynamics related to the perinatal problems, problems in the relationship with the mother and father (the feeling of being sexualized by the father), and identification with the deceased brother.

Autism

Nikolaas Tinbergen (ethologist, Nobel Prize laureate) believed that autism is based on a long-term internal motivational conflict, manifested by the coexistent tendencies to approach and avoid (Tinbergen and Tinbergen 1983). The methods of ethology led him to many observations confirming the conflicting nature of autism, for example, he pointed to the characteristic hand posture that often occurs in autistic children, which looks like a kind of combination of the desire to catch with a lack of confidence to do it.

This theory of motivational conflict corresponds to the observations of Hellinger, who sees in autism the mechanism of withdrawal from the environment as a kind of defense against the impulses stem from identification with the murderer. From the point of view of constellations, behaviors of the autist would be a symptom of a strong internal conflict that seizes the child's emotions and body, making him unable to develop normally.

How can one present the situation of an autistic? He feels as if he were taken out and placed in a strange place. He is so deeply connected with the family past as if he were in it. According to earlier theories, the causes of autism lay in the personality and behavior of the parents, which is false. However, perhaps also the parents, play a role in this regard. The father may not have inner resources to say to the child "You are here."

One's birth is also often an important factor in autism. Probably, many autistic children were delivered in a way that did not let them feel full contact with their mother, which resulted in interrupting the bond with her. This causes—as experiences of representatives show—that the child feels lonely, isolated from everyone, as if he was living in an inhuman world.

A constellation concerning Adrian, a seven-year-old boy, showed the abortions his grandmother had had and the victims who had been probably related to the great-grandfather, a soldier of the Soviet army. Taking this great-grandfather into Adrian's heart—which he did through his representative—proved to be particularly important. Finally, the representative, standing among the family members and the dead, said with joy, "I have a family at last."

When I spoke to Adrian's mother and father before the constellation, they described their families as ordinary, as if not worth mentioning. However, I had a clear feeling that something was hidden, that there were secrets there. It was only during the constellation that Adrian's mother disclosed some facts (such as the abortions, her grandfather's military past, and other). When it was displayed that Adrian was attached to his great-grandfather—or actually wanted him to be fully brought back in the family system—Adrian's parents remembered that the son kept saying "grandfather." Nobody knew why, because no one in their home ever mentioned the grandfathers and he did not know them.

The boy calmed down and laid down next to the representative of one of the deceased persons several times. He also began to recite the alphabet, which in his case was a highly organized and calm behavior. Was he counting the system members and ordering them? I also noticed that while playing with a mobile phone, he began to record the constellation.

Anastasia's constellation concerning her eighteen-year-old autistic daughter, Veronica, casts another light on the complex matter of autism. At one point during the constellation, I asked the client about her own birth. She replied that there were no complications, but that some students were present in the labor room. When I asked about this, we were sitting with our backs together, and I represented "something related to her condition" (drowsiness, weakness, and unwillingness to live).

In the beginning, I did not find the information about the students to be important, however, I found myself imagining a group of people standing opposite, and I said about it to those participating in the constellation. At that point, the client—who spontaneously shared her memories and feelings—said that as a child she was sexually abused several times. A hypothesis came to my mind that the presence of the students was a kind of sexual abuse against the mother. I also said that it seemed that the child had detected the mother's embarrassment and decided that she would not cause an additional problem. I had the thought that the baby had wanted to be born "without touching the mother." When I said about the students standing in front of me, the representative of the client's mother felt that "something was lifted off her shoulders" (a frequent sign that what has been said is true). And the client began to say that she had taken over the shame of other people all her life, that it had been easy to manipulate her when this feeling had been involved.

Later in the constellation, I represented the client's autistic daughter. I felt that I wanted to put my head between her mother's legs to establish a bond this way. Anastasia felt enormous shame. This did not correspond with the situation—the client was an open person and was not ashamed to talk about her aggressive impulses toward her daughter, or about her sexuality, she was also familiar with constellations. Her shame was "that" shame, and it was not directly caused by what was happening during the constellation.

Interestingly, earlier Anastasia had said that she liked to squeeze through, wrestle with someone (which actually happened in the constellation). During the constellation, Anastasia had various feelings about her daughter, including a desire to cut her to pieces, destruct her—which she honestly communicated. She also felt that she would like to die herself, to "rot." After the constellation, she said that she felt something had finally separated from her, as if she had not fully given birth to her daughter before, because some part of her psyche had remained inside her. This was in line with my feeling that the daughter had needed her birth to be completed. The client could now look at her daughter, which earlier, as she said herself, had been difficult for her. The contact with the daughter could become less ambivalent now.

The constellation was very complex. In addition to what I described, it showed that the autistic daughter was identified with the perpetrator (both me and the client built a picture of blood). Anastasia said that the labor and delivery of her daughter, which was extremely difficult, was conducted by "a butcher"—a doctor who cut her unnecessarily and carelessly. There was a vague thread of probably the war (the "Germans"). An important element was also the client's strange weakness, which the daughter seemed to follow (constant drowsiness). All in all, it seemed that in the mind of the autistic daughter many threads merged: the birth of the mother who "did not touch" her mother; the murder of the past; the "butcher" from the labor room; the students; the Germans; the mother's strange drowsiness and weakness; and the archaic and ambivalent relationship with her. It was too much for her to remain mentally healthy. Despite the many interpretative ambiguities of that constellation, it seems to show the etiological multifactorness of autism. It also draws attention to the importance of birth. The thread of transgenerational amplification of the problem occurs here—an "incomplete" birth leads to a more "incomplete" birth in the next generation.

Jack and Madelyn had an autistic, seven-year-old son who was born by caesarean section as their first and only child in the twelfth year of their marriage. A year before our meeting, he uttered his first word, "mother." This happened on the day when during the funeral of an old aunt another relative revealed a family secret—she described the circumstances and the perpetrator of the murder within the family. In the beginning of the constellation, there was a representative of the autistic boy and a representative of "something/someone he was unconsciously bound to." Earlier, the parents had said that the boy behaved as if he had had some invisible companion, as if he had turned to some imaginary figure. In the constellation, the representative of the boy lay down on his side, and the person (he was bound to) was sitting next to him, touching him. I added a representative of Madelyn. As a mother, she had no resources to take care of the child. She was stiff. I set up her mother's representative, and asked Madelyn's representative to lie down on the floor.

It turned out that Madelyn's mother was also bound to something. Madelyn said that when her mother was pregnant with her, her mother's mother (Madelyn's grandmother) died. Madelyn's mother was only 21 years old then. I asked the representative of Madelyn's mother to say in the direction of the chair, representing Madelyn's grandmother now: "What you gave me is enough. Thank you. I know you're with me." After the constellation, Madelyn told me that she had recently taken out her grandmother's photograph from the frame, and on the reverse, there had been the sentences written by her mother: "You left too soon. I've missed you." It was this dynamics of grievance and a sense of lack of support that I noticed in the constellation and helped Madelyn's mother to take a step toward the solution—by expressing through the representative's mouth a thank-you and saying that as much as she got was enough.

When I invited the real parents to enter the constellation, Madelyn wanted to touch or hug her son's representative (a woman), but she shuddered and moved away. She let the father touch her, but she felt better when he took his hand away. She was in her world, bound to someone. I asked Madelyn to stand in front of her mother. Madelyn accepted her mother and stayed in her arms for a longer time. In the end, the boy's representative—extremely deeply immersed in the role—sat down opposite the father. She was shivering, as if trying to say something, fighting with herself. It looked as if she wanted to wake up, get out of a cocoon, or be born. I helped her by suggesting the word "Dad." This was the word she wanted to say. "Da . . .ad," she said, stuttering, to finally say, "Dad." She became more conscious, present.

This constellation also indicates the multiple causality of autism. We can see the coexistence of factors such as homicide in the family and the secret associated with it ("prohibition of speaking"), perinatal problems ("incomplete birth," no early bond with the mother), transgenerational aggregation of the problem (the problem of the bond with the mother during the birth of the autist's mother, then the problem with her own child). The boy remained in his own world because he was not fully born mentally. Perhaps, if there is a lack of bond with the parents in the earliest possible period of life, the child's psyche is particularly focused on searching for a bond with someone from the depths of the system, probably someone dead. This kind of relationship is a kind of substitutive relationship (the child is strongly bound to such a person, sometimes he can be represented by the child's favorite toy or some object that the child holds on to). The mother and the perinatal events were very important in the cited constellation, but the way to the outside world was the father. It was in his relationship with him that the son began to wake up. It is likely that the father's role is similar in many other cases of autism.

Neurotic Disorders

Systemic constellations have much to offer in therapy of neuroses. Serious therapeutic difficulties occur only in the case of obsessive-compulsive disorder, because this disorder consists in a deep transformation of the structure of the self (Janus 2019, 43–63). In such cases, the whole personality is subject to the obsessive way of responding. Besides his obsessions, the affected person "does not exist" because he has no sphere independent of the obsessive pattern of functioning.

A constellation can interrupt obsessive thinking for people whose obsessive-compulsive disorder is not severe, but for people with severe neurosis, it does not work. The obsessive self is a kind of entirety without gaps, which is why it is not able to accept the radically new knowledge offered by a constellation. The individual would first have to agree to a severe disturbance of his balance, and obsessive-compulsive disorder is precisely a strenuous attempt to maintain a kind of balance, or rather permanent mental immobility. Still, constellations can contribute a lot to therapy of obsessive-compulsive patients, showing that their neurotic behaviors are formed in a broader context. This concerns the events that involve death and guilt, shed blood. Therefore, during constellations, representatives start to wipe their hands. The same behaviors occur in patients, because compulsive hand washing is probably the most common compulsion.

Obsessive-compulsive disorder usually results from a legacy of guilt. Someone—a son, grandson, or great-grandson—feels a stain on him that does not actually concern him. It may be caused by a murder that has been concealed. The image of hereditary guilt in obsessive-compulsive disorder corresponds with psychoanalytical concepts. The case of a patient with obsessive-compulsive disorder (Ernst Lanzer known as the Rat Man) analyzed by Freud concerned the son's imaginary attempts to deal with his father's embezzlement and debt.[1] Perhaps there was some earlier and more dramatic guilt involved, not only the one he mentioned to Freud.

Brian was obsessively afraid that he would lose one of his sons. He was constantly looking back and checking if they were nearby. When he opened the door slightly for a moment, he had an irrational feeling that his sons had run outside, and he had a compulsion to make sure that they were still at home. He had even more bizarre fears that someone might have switched one of his sons. When he lost sight of one of them for a moment, he later asked him questions or examined his birthmarks to make sure that he was definitely his son. He had to track everything—as he said himself—"frame by frame," and each gap caused his anxiety. For example, when he could not see when his son changed clothes, he was worried about what might have happened during that time. He was intelligent, sensitive, and well aware that his obsessions were absurd.

Let us now look into the structure of such obsessiveness. There is something wrong here with space-time (Janus 2019, 54). Brian did not seem to trust his perception and saw reality as unstable—therefore, although it was impossible, he was afraid that the child had flashed through the door gap in a second, that a magical switch had taken place, that something significant had happened in half a minute. Did Brian live in our space-time or in another one?

I started to represent—as I put it—his "part that wants to tell us something through the symptoms." I slightly bent and lifted my left leg, then clenched my hands, tensed the muscles of the face, shrank in myself. There was much effort and suffering in it. Then I lay on my side. I asked Brian how he felt. He said he felt very tired at first, and now he could rest. I felt so too. I said I wanted to sleep. Brian said that he often felt sleepy, that he calmed down when he went to bed, then he no longer felt that overwhelming responsibility. I remembered that he told me during the first meeting that he had been born with a shorter leg (I thought it was the left leg, because I slightly bent it, but the client informed me that the right leg was shorter—then I realized that actually I felt that way, I bent my left leg, because it seemed longer to me).

After some time, I turned on my back and stretched my right hand to the side, as if looking for someone. After a while, I had the impression—which I let turn into a visualization—that a person appeared from this side, approached me, kneeled close, and put a hand on me. I told Brian about it. Brian replied that he had a childhood memory that kept coming back to him: he wakes up at night and calls his mother, the mother comes and he tells her about his fear of death. I think I was precisely going through that event and that state. I told the client that a child is not generally afraid of his own death, but of *some* death—the death he heard about, he saw, or anticipated. At the end, I felt the energy to get up, and we embraced—Brian integrated the split-off part and its life force. So someone's death was the point here, and Brian was unconsciously connected with it. It kept him off the normal space-time completely. He said, for example, that sometimes when he walked down the street, he felt as if he had hovered over himself, as if he had not been in his body. He was connected with someone's death and was, therefore, absent himself.

Obsessiveness and death? They were linked by Jacques Lacan, who maintained that the obsessive-compulsive neurotic is absorbed in the question: "Am I dead or alive?" (Fink 1997, 126).

NOTE

1. The thought of rats became part of Ernst Lanzer's neurosis after he had been told during the military maneuvers about a kind of torture that involved pushing a rat into the anus.

Chapter 8

The Systemic Context of Psychoses

DELUSIONS AND HALLUCINATIONS IN SCHIZOPHRENIA

Productions or Perceptions?

In September 1939, Jacob Moreno began a therapeutic psychodrama with an immigrant from Germany, referred to as Karl L. The patient was psychotic and claimed that he was the real Adolf Hitler. Moreno asked his trainees in psychodrama to enact "Goebbels," "Goering," and other notables. The therapy was successful, and after 18 sessions, Karl L. had his mustache shaved off, realizing that he was not Hitler at all. However, the most interesting was the course of therapy itself. Moreno wrote:

> He seemed to know everything in advance; many things he presented on the stage came very close to what actually took place years later. He appeared to have a special sense for fitting himself into moods and decisions which were made thousands of miles apart from him. In fact, at times we speculated whether he, the patient, was not the real Hitler and the other in Germany his double. We had the strange experience of feeling the real Hitler among us, working desperately on finding a solution for himself. [. . .] At other times, he portrayed moods of great desperation, feelings that he had failed and that the Reich would be conquered by its enemies. In one of these moods, he stepped upon the stage and declared that the time had come for him to end his life. He asked all the Gestapo leaders who filled the audience—from Goering, Goebbels, Ribbentrop, Hess, down to the last man—to die with him. [. . .] He shot himself in front of the audience. (Moreno and Moreno 2011, 196–97)

Moreno also noted the patient's words: "'What's the matter with me? [. . .] Will this torture never end? Is it real or is it a dream?'" (Moreno and Moreno 2011, 197). It suggests that Karl L. had some distance to his experiences. Was he really connected to Adolf Hitler in a way? According to the patterns of the dominant psychology, this would obviously be impossible. And yet, a well-known psychiatrist, Ronald David Laing, describing a schizophrenic female patient who manifested delusions of influence, expresses his doubt about the current understanding of the nature of interpersonal interactions:

> Now, in general, the nature of the reciprocal influences that persons do and can exert on one another is rather obscure. [. . .] Certainly it would be easier to discuss Maya's preoccupation with this issue if clearer ideas existed among the sane population on what does and can happen in this respect. (Laing and Esterson 2017, 11)

In turn, psychoanalyst Sándor Ferenczi wrote:

> I do not exclude the possibility that delusional productions contain more objective reality than we have assumed until now. From the very beginning I was inclined to think that the hallucinations of the insane, or at least a part of them, are not imaginings but real perceptions, stemming from the environment and from the psyches of other human beings, which are accessible to them—precisely because of their psychologically motivated hypersensitivity—whereas normal people, focusing only on immediate matters of direct concern to them, remain unaffected. (Ferenczi 1995, 58)

One can sometimes observe a strange ability of schizophrenics to read unconscious messages and their extrasensory access to knowledge of other people. What the more attentive psychiatrists observe is, primarily, the knowledge of people from the patient's immediate environment, physicians, and other patients. Listening to the seemingly incoherent speech of schizophrenics, one can sometimes discover that they are aware of some undisclosed aspects of someone's personality or life. When, for example, a psychiatrist has just had an argument with his wife, they can talk about it in an indirect or symbolic way, and when he is afraid of something, they too can experience an increased level of anxiety.

However, I think it is much more important that psychotics have access to hidden knowledge of their family members. A psychotic, Georg, said his grandfather was evil and did something terrible, although he did not know anything about the grandfather's life. His delusions were focused around that imagined evil of the grandfather. The constellation suggested that the grandfather might have tried to kill his unborn son, who was eventually born handicapped. It seems that Georg knew this without the constellation. There are many similar examples.

What are psychoses? They are deep mental disorders, characterized by the occurrence of delusions and hallucinations, disturbances of consciousness, significant disturbances of emotions and mood as well as disturbances of thinking and social functioning. These mental disorders are the deepest of all, and they disorganize life the most. Psychoses primarily include paranoia, schizophrenia, and schizoaffective disorders, but deep depression and bipolar disorder may also have psychotic aspects.

With regard to psychoses Hellinger said:

> My insights into psychoses go very far. And many suffering people could be helped. But these insights are often strongly opposed by psychiatrists. And also resisted by the families of the sick. Why? Because deep down, at a deeply unconscious level, they are happy that someone suffers from psychosis. They feel relieved because if the patient did not suffer from psychosis, someone else would have to suffer from it. (Hellinger and Nehrebecki 2012, 171)[1]

The fact that families often, in some way, oppose recovery of the patient is widely observed by psychotherapists. It is also not difficult to see that most psychiatrists "take over" psychotics because they justify the meaning of their profession. This also frequently involves separating such patients from other forms of help.

Hellinger's insights concern the identification of psychotic persons with murderers and their victims. He also observed that schizophrenic patients identify with people of the opposite sex (Hellinger 2001, 370). The latter is partly confirmed by the observations of psychoanalysts, who point to the characteristic feminization of male psychotics, although they consider it to be caused by other factors (Fink 1997, 98–99).

Thanks to what we experience as representatives, we can probably better understand symptoms of psychosis. During constellations, we employ what I call spontaneous visualizations, which in most cases turn out to be accurate information about the client's system. We "see" the lying dead, we "see" that the imagined person moves away or closer, we see that there are many people involved in a given case. Obviously, these are not clear and spectacular images. Their visual layer is poor, but they express rudimentary facts about the family.

Can similar phenomena underlie hallucinations? My experiences with psychotic people suggest that they can. I believe that nonpsychotic people, including psychiatrists, imagine visual hallucinations in a simplified way—always simply as visual images. They reach this conclusion based on the patient's account, but primarily on their own experiences with seeing (Janus 2019, 194). However, the patient is not able to fully describe with words how he "sees" and their own experiences are too poor to make them able to get an adequate picture of this kind of experience. Probably, patients often have only a feeling of someone's presence and not clear images. Thanks to the knowledge provided by systemic constellations, we understand that there may be different degrees of "seeing." We do not need to insist that hallucinations are merely a result of the projection of the patient's inner world, but we know that they may carry knowledge of nonsubjective aspects of reality, for example, knowledge of specific people from the system.

Auditory hallucinations are another phenomenon. They occur more frequently than visual hallucinations and are actually a common human experience (Watkins 2008). Can some of these phenomena have the same background as—known to people who take part in constellations—the words and sentences that come spontaneously to their heads? Sometimes in an almost audible form. Perhaps some of these voices are productions of the psyche, for example, commenting voices that only report what the person does. However, other ones may result from telepathic and systemic influences. So their final shape may be the resultant of telepathy, "information from the ancestors" and the individual functioning of one's own psyche.

Delusions of Influence

Psychoses are characterized by the occurrence of delusions, which psychiatry defines as false and unshakable beliefs. Interestingly, however, most of delusions involve some kind of influence on the patient or his influence on others. And so there are delusions concerning poisoning, harming one's reputation, being eavesdropped, peeped, or persecuted in other ways, as well as delusional beliefs in own ability to influence others, make them fall sick, stutter, flush. This category also includes delusions of reference, that is, the patient's conviction that the world revolves around him, so they write about him in newspapers or speak on television.

Among all kinds of delusions, a large group are those that refer to paranormal influences. They occur mainly in paranoid schizophrenia and play a significant role in the diagnosis of this disease. Already Emil Kraepelin, who developed the detailed concept of dementia praecox (the term was first used by Arnold Pick), maintained that one of the most characteristic features of this disease is "the feeling that the patient knows the thoughts of other people" (Greyson 1977, 184). Eugen Bleuler, who renamed *dementia praecox* as *schizophrenia*, argued that "the feelings of thoughts being heard and transmitted" to others are "almost pathognomonic" of this disease (Greyson 1977, 184). Kurt Schneider, the author of a weighty diagnostic system, also considered this kind of beliefs and sensations of patients as phenomena specific of schizophrenia (Greyson 1977, 184). These include the beliefs that one's thoughts are inserted into one's mind, withdrawn, or broadcasted and heard by others, experience of influences playing on the body, "made" feelings, impulses, and acts (Crowhurst and Coles 1989, 239). The ICD-10 diagnostic manual mentions, inter alia: "thought echo; thought insertion or withdrawal; thought broadcasting; delusional perception and delusions of control; influence or passivity" (ICD-10, n.d.).

So schizophrenics maintain that their thoughts or feelings are broadcasted to others, they are convinced that someone inserts or takes their thoughts away, that someone controls their mind or body. Other people cease to be separate and in a way mingle with them. The boundaries between the patient's ego and the environment get blurred.

Mainstream psychiatry has not believed these sensations for years, considering them to be productive symptoms, in other words—morbid creations that have nothing to do with reality. However, the knowledge provided by systemic constellations requires that the suffering of schizophrenics be examined with greater attention. Even the fact that their experiences are so similar is thought-provoking. People with schizophrenia claim that they have electronic chips in their heads, that they are controlled by radio waves, by aliens, or associations of telepaths. Why do different people invariably talk about the same things—about influences on their thoughts, about breaking into their heads, about remote control? Why do their brains not produce a whole kaleidoscope of bizarre reactions, but these repetitive patterns?

Thanks to constellations, we know that extrasensory influences of one psyche on another one really exist, which makes it possible for us to look at schizophrenia more openly and extensively. This does not mean we have to admit that what schizophrenic patients say is true. However, we should consider whether psychosis uncovers something of the essence of the mind and interpersonal relations. Perhaps in schizophrenia, apart from an extreme disturbance of one's sense of identity, peculiarities, and difficulties in social functioning, what is also brought to light are transpersonal influences that function in the lives of healthy people too but are not as directly experienced by them.

This view was represented by psychiatrist Jan Ehrenwald (Ehrenwald 1947, 121 et seq.). He believed that paranoid patients, focused on allegedly being persecuted, have telepathic access to the sadistic and aggressive levels of the psyche of those around them. This causes that—in a sense—they really have something to be afraid of. Whereas, schizophrenic patients are focused on less specific, more generalized, although hidden too, levels of other people's psyches. Ehrenwald cited many examples that indicated the telepathic abilities of his patients. At the same time, he believed that external psychological influence is only one of the elements forming the picture of psychosis, next to the influence of the patient's own unconscious content.

Ehrenwald believed that the original symbiotic relationship with the mother is of a telepathic nature, which in the course of development is transformed into ordinary communication. However, a child who has not successfully gone through the separation-individuation stage, which means he has not separated his own psychic processes from those of his mother, continues to a certain extent the original and symbiotic ways of communication. He may therefore be vulnerable to the mother's telepathic intrusions (Greyson 1977, 185). This would be the case for psychotics.

Also psychiatrist Jule Eisenbud found that a significant part of our behaviors and affects, both morbid and normal, cannot be "meaningfully patternized without the aid of a hypothesis such as that of telepathic interaction and intercommunication between individuals" (Eisenbud 1952, 51).

Christopher, a twenty-year-old suffering from schizophrenia, felt that his friends from his childhood and adolescence tried to break into his mind, take control over his psyche (in the past, they tried to dominate him, sometimes they were aggressive and laughed at him). Christopher's suffering lasted for many years, and of course, none of the psychiatrists took the problem of his friends attacking his brain seriously. For me, it was clear that Christopher described something that he experienced. Even without recognizing the possibility of this kind of influence, it was necessary to work with what he felt. Christopher told me he felt that a friend wanted him to "submit" in this remote way. He also claimed that in childhood his grandfather had influenced him with words, and his grandmother had done it rather "psychologically," that now they "were sitting" in his head and he could not get rid of their influence. When he espoused one political party, he was ("in the head") attacked by the members of the competing party. He maintained that most people were strong, and he was weak, hence that constant influence on him.

During an individual constellation I stood as his friend Z. I asked Christopher to say a few sentences like "I'm letting you go" to the friend. At first, Christopher tried to reject the friend, but I encouraged him to look at him without fear and say goodbye to him rather than chase him away. We worked with the figures of his grandmother and grandfather in a similar form. Christopher reacted intensely during the constellation, and after it was finished, he said that I had helped him a lot, that now it was much better. This condition persisted when I talked to him a few months later.

THE SYSTEMIC-PSYCHODYNAMIC CONCEPT OF SCHIZOPHRENIA

There is a fact that seems to support psychotics' great focus on influences from others. They usually turn away from the family and become hostile or indifferent toward it. Strangers often turn out to be extremely significant to them, while the family ceases to matter. Why does this happen? It looks as if the inner turning away from the father, mother, and family results in opening to influences from other people—real and imagined influences. A compensation mechanism is probable here, as if the psyche did not tolerate such detachment from the family and brought in some kind of substitutes in place of the significant figures. Psychotic people are interested in global and cosmic matters and magnify the trivial actions of others, perceiving them as deeply meaningful for their own lives. They have their heads in the clouds and are unable to accept the existential and grounding meaning of their ancestors and family.

However, referring to one's mother, father, and members of the family system is visible in psychosis. It often starts with considerations about one's childhood, family, and one's place in it. Later, this image gets replaced by general and more philosophical or religious considerations. Sometimes the two processes are almost parallel, and the family threads are immediately transformed into symbolic images. This can be understood as a defense mechanism that presents the most difficult and incomprehensible threads in the form of content that is easier to bear and expressible.

Based on the observations of other authors and systemic constellations, I distinguish several possible mechanisms that form the picture of schizophrenia. Experiencing mysterious influences from the environment may be due to the following:

1. Altered perception, where the stimuli that are normally peripheral or unnoticed come to the fore, as it were, flooding the schizophrenic's mind;
2. Nonfunctioning of the mechanism of repression—the content that is normally unconscious becomes significantly important in the individual's consciousness;
3. Increased sensitivity to projections and nonverbal messages from people in the individual's environment;
4. Telepathic sensitivity to other people's minds;
5. Increased sensitivity (awareness) to information contained in the family field.

Points (1) and (2) are conventional explanations concerning the individual psyche. They relate to the schizophrenic's increased sensitivity to external and internal stimuli. Explanation (3) is an intermediate between thinking in terms of ordinary sensory perception and ESP. This stems from the fact that such concepts of psychoanalysis as "projective identification," when considered in an unbiased way, refer to rudimentary telepathic processes (Brottman 2011, chap. 5). Therefore, the reception of the hetero-psychic material, and thus telepathic sensitivity, plays an important role in the formation of schizophrenic feelings, delusions, and general functioning of the patient. However, the telepathic aspects of schizophrenia are only one of the elements of the general blurring of the ego boundaries and the specific opening of schizophrenics to hidden, typically unconscious, aspects of reality (Janus 2019, 122 et seq.).

The general "openness" of schizophrenics causes them to react to the influence from the family field in a different, more direct way. In their case, the mechanism of systemic-psychodynamic transduction (the concept of systemic-psychodynamic transduction is described in chapter 11) is of a different character—its processes reach the consciousness of the subject to a greater extent.

Ultimately, the picture of schizophrenia is shaped by the hetero- and auto-psychic influences as well as by the sensitivity of the sick. Here, we can refer to the words of Ehrenwald, who believes that schizophrenia "is the result of the intrusion into the patient's consciousness of primitive material from *both* the auto-psychic and the hetero-psychic sphere, and his individual reaction to this alarming experience" (Ehrenwald 1947, 150). Based on the conclusions drawn from systemic constellations, we must consider not the random and changeable telepathic influences, but the permanent influence of the family field to be the most important among hetero-psychic influences.

The mechanism may be so that the schizophrenic becomes partly aware of, for example, the hidden attitude of the parents, family secrets, and awkward facts that have been "swept under the carpet" in his family life. These perceptions become possible both through telepathic channels and through the influence of the family field. The latter constantly "screens" a "film" to our mind about the most important events related to the family (it is this "screening" and "watching" that I define as systemic-psychodynamic transduction). We must remember that every person is influenced by this process from birth or even from the prenatal period. Schizophrenia is caused both by the clarity of this film (which, in accordance with Hellinger's statements and my own experience, contains drastic "scenes" related to a murder or a threat to life), and by the schizophrenic's increased sensitivity. These two factors in a way form the initial process of psychosis, which we can define as an opening phase. The second phase is the phase of defense and projection. The schizophrenic must do something about the conflicting psychic material that floods him. In order to do so, he distances himself from his family and from what is ordinary and concrete. He delves into general, pseudo-political, or religious considerations so characteristic of schizophrenics. In this phase, strangers, such as Doctor Flechsig in the well-known case of Daniel Paul Schreber (Schreber 2000), become excessively meaningful to him. However, the crucial thing, which hits the patient's mind with the greatest force, that is, the parents' inner attitudes and transgenerational factors, remains hidden. Schreber began chapter 3. of his *Memoirs*—probably the most interesting one for us—with the following words:

> I will first consider some events concerning *other members of my family*, which may possibly in some way be related to the presumed soul murder; these are all

more or less mysterious, and can hardly be explained in the light of usual human experience. (Schreber 2000, 43)

Unfortunately, these words are followed by emptiness—as this very chapter did not appear in print. Probably at the request of some members of Schreber's family. So both judge Schreber as well as the psychiatrists and psychoanalysts trying to understand him, were left with what was less important.

OTHER PSYCHOTIC STATES

Paranoia

Christine's delusions referred to the impact of electromagnetic waves on her health and the negative actions of her husband. During many years of treatment, she received various diagnoses ranging from depression, through schizoaffective disorder, to paranoid schizophrenia.[2] She complained mainly about severe headaches, which she associated with the impact of mobile phones, and the environment's unfriendly attitude toward her.

Her psychotherapy lasted several years. As a result, the nagging pain sensations disappeared, and her general mood and ability to function in everyday life improved. Christine was able to take care of her affairs and health (earlier, when she had been submitted to psychiatric treatment and had taken neuroleptics, she had got very fat and her somatic problems had not been treated properly), she renewed her contacts with the living family members, she was able to enter into conflict-free relations with people who provided various services (which had been very problematic before), she felt stronger and regained faith in the future. Her delusional attitude did not disappear, but it no longer disorganized her life.

The psychoanalytical sessions were the most important part of her psychotherapy, but systemic constellations I facilitated at the beginning of the therapy played an important role. Because Christine perceived her husband as a persecutor,[3] and her main suffering was persistent headaches and numbness, I put a piece of paper in front of her, on which she had written "symptoms," and another one with the word "husband." When I stood on the "symptoms" sheet, the client said that the numbness she had felt, suddenly disappeared (which is a characteristic and frequent phenomenon that occurs when some suffering is represented). I asked her to say how she felt about the "symptoms" (that is, me as a representative):

C: Something bad. They want to do something bad to me, like a thug, now I see you this way—evil in your eyes. But I don't think you're like that.

Then I stood on the piece of paper with the word "husband."
C: A thug too. He wants to harm me.

I asked the client to write "mom" on another sheet and put it in a row with the other sheets. I stood on this piece of paper telling Christine that I was representing her mother now. Here are some of the sentences that were said then:

T: What do you feel?
C: I feel that she wants to do something bad to me. She's evil too. Yes, she also wants to do something bad to me.
T: Your mom doesn't have bad feelings for you.
C: Yes, I'm angry with her for dying. She left me.
T: "You're to blame, you died so soon."
C: Maybe she wants to take me so that I don't suffer here.
T: She didn't leave you, she died. But she is also with you all the time.
C: I see that tears spring to your eyes (it was true), to my eyes too. Maybe I was angry with her because she'd died, because I thought she'd left me.
T: Please say, "Mom, thank you. For the time you were here."
C: Yes, thank you, Mom, for being with me then and looking at me all the time.

Another constellation. The client spoke about the malice she experienced from the people around, and about the fear of her hearing in court: "I don't know how it's going to be in this court, how I'll survive it. I hope I won't start to behave in a strange way. They'll take me to hospital and finish me off there. You'll see, it will be so."

I put a rug in front of Christine and asked who was lying on it.

C: My husband. Dearest mother!
T: "Dearest mother." Anyone else?
C: My children . . . grandmother . . . grandparents . . . Mary . . . all these people . . . you . . . people . . . doctor D . . . my mother, father.
T: Please, look at the mother, she is lying here. Now I will represent her (I lay down on the rug).

In the further part of this constellation, I suggested that the client say "Thank you" and take her mother into the heart. The client thanked and felt the mother in her heart (she said that she had a place in her heart close to the child she had aborted). She asked her mother to protect her and make her life fall into place. This sentence, however, weakened the thank-you—I could clearly feel that it contained a hidden grievance against the mother. That is why I asked the client again to thank the mother. I also asked her to take her mother's hand, because she did not have to be afraid of her.

C: There is some fear.
T (Mother): Chrissie, you also have strength.
C: Yes, I feel it, I have strength, I can still do a lot.
T: Please bow to your mom. "Thank you, Mom."
C: Thank you, Mom.

After the constellation, we had a few minutes' break and the client went to the bathroom. When she returned, she said that after leaving the bathroom, when she was passing near the place where I had been lying, she felt for a moment "this smell of death." Then, in a rather nervous way, she started talking about the strange text messages and danger again. I consider her behavior as a negative reaction to a possible change in her inner attitude. It had occurred many times before. The function of this reaction is not clear. There are basically two possibilities: either it is a kind of mental inertia or this reaction indicates unknown aspects of the client's problem.

When in the next constellation I stood as the client's "life" (which we can understand also as her "previous life," "the one that she lived until now"), she could not simply accept it; she had some objections. She could not take life because—in her opinion—it was destroyed by other people, it was not what she wanted. She constantly held grudge against the others, which she had to mention as soon as she was just about to say the formula: "I accept you, you are mine." Accepting her life with no "buts" would equal withdrawing delusional projections, at least for a moment. Accepting one's life is recognizing and accepting this dimension of existence in which one is a pure subject, belongs just to oneself. It is recognizing the aspect of one's individuality and separation from others. The client could not do it. She had to be connected with others through persecution on their part (this kind of transitivism—peculiar mixing of the subject and the other—was manifested through her tendency to say what she saw in me, not what she felt for me as a representative).

Only after over a year of therapy did Christine mention that she had a baby sister who died in the first weeks after her birth, probably infected by her sick mother. This information was obviously very important. In the next systemic exercise, I asked her to write on several sheets of paper what age she was in the important moments of her life, from the present to the past. She was supposed to speak about the event, and write only the age she was at the time. So we had a few sheets referring to such situations as the termination of therapy with the psychiatrist, who unsuccessfully treated her for about 20 years, her son's wedding, her first stay in a mental hospital, primary school, and finally the stay with the mother's parents at the age of three.

I put the sheets on the floor in a straight line one after another so that the sheet with the age of "3" lay right next to an armchair. Then I asked the client to stand on the first sheet, then on the second, and so on. In this way, she flashed back in her memory, feelings also came to her. This stage was intended only to prepare her for the main process. When the client stood on the sheet "3," I asked her to say nothing. Then I said that she was going back to the age of two, when her sister still lived, and asked her to sit in the armchair. At the same time I informed her that now I represented her sister—at this point, I squatted by the chair. I started to breathe quickly, as if I was panting in a fever. Christine said that she felt her sister around the womb, the sister was choking because no one helped her. Then, she said she felt her in the neck. At the end—in the heart. She said her sister had died, but she lived in her. She added that if her sister lived, it would be different, she would help her, she said, "It's a pity she died."

Representing the sister, I felt anxious all the time, but I eventually calmed down. The sentences of strength I proposed were, inter alia: "You died when I was a child. You were even smaller," "You are in my heart," "I could not do anything," "I leave your fate with you." When I suggested these sequences I realized that, for example, the sentence "I leave your fate with you" would not or could not be fully accepted. The bond between the client and her sister was of a different nature, and this sentence was not fully adequate. Christine even said something like she "was" her sister. She finally felt calm, unburdened, and hopeful (before this happened, she had had headaches—probably the same as those associated with the sense of persecution). In this constellation, one can see the cooccurrence of identification and rivalry, love as well as fear and rejection. Christine identified with her sister; she probably identified with her mother too (feeling her sister in the womb area). She feared and rejected them at the same time. These dynamics related to her family were the basis of her projections onto other people.[4]

Delusional Reactions

Besides deep psychotic states, characterized by bizarre beliefs and lack of criticism, there are less personality-disrupting states. I mean distrustful attitudes, anticipating bad intentions of others, and guesses about their intrigues and conspiracies. Sometimes these types of states can be temporary and accompany severe interpersonal stress or traumatic life events.

During the initial conversation, Ann told an extensive story about intrigues, malice, and injustice in her family. Her grandmother's sisters reportedly took possession of some property and the aunt reportedly took something from the mother. The other aunts told other people something that had a negative impact on the family. Among other things, about the grandmother—namely, that "she was sick." I asked if it was a mental illness, which the client confirmed.

Ann constantly said, "They . . . us . . . ," and all this was filled with conflict and persecution. I asked who told her those stories. Ann knew most of them from her mother, although she swore that she had also experienced this or that herself. Even before the constellation, I said that I did not believe in these stories. I said that of course, there are greedy aunts and family members that may be hard to bear, but this story takes place mainly in her head, it is a kind of fairy tale that she tells herself and others.

In the constellation, the mother ran away from the grandmother, being afraid of her and wanting to take refuge with her father. Ann's representative did not feel so much fear, but she also felt better by her father. It was about something from the distant past; when I set it up (I put a sheet of paper that represented it), the grandmother calmed down. Before, she had only been interested in saving her daughter, but it caused that the latter feared even more.

This example corresponds with my other observations, which I could express with the sentence: "Paranoia comes from the mother." At least in many cases. Here, we had the mother, terrified since childhood, who tried hard to "protect" her daughter from bad people, which in fact came down to transmitting her own fear. Peace could be found by the father.

Patricia came to me after the man she knew had sued her for harassment and threats. She had had a nonsexual relationship with him, as I understood it, and had sent him hundreds of text messages for several months. The client claimed that he provoked her and she could not refrain from sending the messages to him. She described the man's character, as well as his impact on her, using the vocabulary of psychoanalysis: she spoke about the split-off parts of his self, deficits, projective identification, containing, and early traumas. The text messages contained interpretations of his behavior, by which she tried to "get through to him," believing that he was not aware of what was happening to him.

Indeed, Patricia's concept of her interaction with the man was coherent, and I was inclined to agree that much of what she said about the man's character was a relevant observation. It was obvious, however, that I was dealing with delusions.

Because Patricia claimed that the man was the essence of her problem, I set up her representative and a representative of that man. It was not surprising to me that neither he nor the client's representative were interested in each other. The man stepped aside and looked blankly out the window, and the client's representative said that he did not interest her. The whole constellation was multithreaded, but the essence of the problem was Patricia's relationship with her grandfather, who had died before her birth. The constellation revealed that the grandfather (and partly grandmother) was particularly bound to some deceased—something dramatic had happened, possibly related to the war or a murder. Patricia was strongly bound to him and took on herself those difficult stories. The paranoid projection was a defense mechanism, a kind of reaction to the transgenerational trauma.

Bipolar Disorder

Bipolar disorder is characterized by alternating mania and depression. Bert Hellinger considers incest to be its root. However, the systemic picture of the disease can be complex.

Michael's father suffered from a severe form of manic-depressive disorder and could not participate in the constellation. The father's father (Michael's grandfather) killed a woman in a car accident. As a representative of Michael's father, I looked up and reached my hand out there, then I hit the wall with my hands. I felt anxiety, a kind of confusion, and I was afraid of the father's representative. Then I started walking very quickly around the chair representing the dead woman. I felt an erotic fascination, mixed with fears. I asked if the accident had happened when the father was small and learned that he had been about two years old. I asked whether the father's mother had been absent in his early life. Michael said that after the accident she had defended her husband from prison and that she had fallen into depression. So it was likely that the mother was emotionally unavailable and that the movement of love was interrupted. Michael also remembered that his father had had a video cassette with a pornographic film including both sex and homicide. He said he was also interested in something like that. The representative of the grandfather who had caused the accident showed no interest in the deceased. His son took this interest on himself. It seemed that the child formed a special type of unconscious relationship with the deceased.

Perhaps in manic states—that occur in bipolar disorder—the bond with the deceased usually takes a form that evokes euphoria in the sick person. This would correspond to Hellinger's opinion that mania is identification with someone who is "in heaven," so in a rather pleasant state. In this case, there was an erotic aspect, and the deceased woman could be a substitute for the inaccessible mother. This in turn would correspond with the element of incest in bipolar disorder indicated by Ruppert; here, however, not in the form of a real act.

PREGNANCY AND CHILDBIRTH AND PSYCHOSIS

Walter was twenty-eight years old. When he was seventeen, just after the death of his eleven-year-old brother (he was found hung, but it was probably an accident), he fell into depression, started to have fears and visions. He used various drugs, took Prozac for years, he took haloperidol and other neuroleptics for more than a year, which he recently stopped because he felt better. He was afraid of being among people and therefore could not work. He came to the constellation workshop with his mother.

At the beginning, I set up Walter's representative and representatives of his mother and father. The father "wasn't to the liking" of Walter's representative, the son wanted him to move away. I set up "something that concerned Walter and was important." The mother's representative immediately felt that it had something to do with her. Then I asked about Walter's birth. His mother said that it was very difficult—the child choked, which threatened his life. Since then I defined this "something" as his "birth." Later I also added "death." "Death" approached Walter, they embraced each other, then it moved away. At the end, I put the "birth" in front of the client and the representatives of his parents. Walter spontaneously crouched and grabbed the "birth" by the hands. After some time, I asked him to stand up. When he knelt by the "birth," he was calm, when he stood up, he became scared. I said, "Look over there (at the "birth") and say: 'You have a place in my heart, and I'm alive. I've lived from the beginning. From the very beginning. And I'm still alive." Walter calmed down completely and brightened.

Walter's problem was that he did not believe in his successful birth. He did not feel like he was fully alive. Later, in his psyche there was probably a kind of accumulation of his birth trauma and the shocks of deaths in the family, especially the death of his brother. These were probably important factors triggering his psychosis. *Nota bene*, the relationship between schizophrenia and perinatal difficulties was also reported in statistical studies (Cannon, Jones, and Murray 2002).

John was a promising musician, but he gave up his studies. He appeared to be on the verge of psychosis. He had a particularly ambivalent relationship with his mother. In the initial phase of the constellation John's representative was the only defined person. The other three persons were brought in gradually and without me assigning them a specific identity. Later, it turned out that one of them was probably John's mother and the other—as could be inferred from the constellation—was his older brother. The identity of the third person remained unknown.

John's representative was confused, he walked between his mother and the unknown person, saying that there was "part of him" in both places (the unknown person seemed to be the client's unborn twin, it was not clear, but when I looked at the representative of the unknown person, I had the impression that I saw someone "not fully developed," disabled).

When I represented John's brother, strange words came to my mind: "She wanted to kill us." They were addressed to the person who later turned out to be the mother. A few days after the constellation, I invited John's mother and asked her about the course of her pregnancy. She said that there were no major difficulties, but after a while she admitted that she did not want this baby. I asked her to sit down comfortably, close her eyes, go back in her mind to the time when she was pregnant and say to the baby: "I accept you." Then she began to cry and said that there was something else—she wanted to miscarry and for that purpose she jumped a lot. She also confessed that she did not want her first son because she was going to leave her husband. I suggested that she imagine her children and say to each of them: "I accept you." I also told her to reject any guilt. John's mental functioning was most probably a reaction to the prenatal threat he had experienced. He did not suffer physical harm, but felt the threatening context in which he was born.

NOTES

1. Quotation translated from Polish.
2. This diagnostic chaos is not unusual in psychiatry and illustrates its cognitive crisis lasting for years.
3. Later, it turned out that her image of the husband was true to a considerable degree, and he himself probably had traits of paranoid personality disorder.
4. In his early text *Family Complexes in the Formation of the Individual* (1938), Jacques Lacan referred to the complex of intrusion, which we could also call the complex of siblings. He argued that the reaction to siblings born in one's early childhood could be a matrix that shapes paranoia.

Chapter 9

Systemic Dynamics in Somatic Diseases

SYSTEMIC PSYCHOSOMATICS

When we address the psychological determinants of somatic diseases, we enter the field of psychosomatics. The Chicago Seven psychosomatic diseases, described by Franz Alexander, include bronchial asthma, peptic ulcer, rheumatoid arthritis, hyperthyroidism, ulcerative colitis, essential hypertension, and atopic dermatitis. Psychosomatic diseases also include eating disorders, migraines, various autoimmune diseases, sometimes pain and some convulsive states, or paralyses, which are referred to as somatization or conversion. The cause of psychosomatic diseases is said to lie "in the head," that is, in the individual mind. However, from the point of view of constellations, this issue looks different. Hellinger says:

> In today's medicine, there is a view that diseases have psychological roots. But this is not entirely true. There is discussion about psychosomatic diseases, which would mean that diseases show something of the psyche. For example, if a person is angry with someone, it is manifested in his body. In a way, it actually happens. But disease cannot be reduced to psychological causes alone. Disease is caused by disorder. (Hellinger and Nehrebecki 2012, 21)[1]

Hellinger says that "there is nothing individual about disease," which emphasizes that the nonindividual factors are crucial in our diseases. So constellations build another type of psychosomatics—systemic psychosomatics. Our body is influenced not only by the conscious or unconscious part of the mind, but also by what I define as extraconsciousness, that is, by systemic and transgenerational dynamics.

Practicing systemic constellations leads to the amazing conclusion that most diseases are psychosomatic, in the aforementioned sense. I was initially reluctant to accept it because it seemed to me that only a small group of diseases could have systemic roots. After all, the body is a complicated mechanism, and mechanisms unfortunately fail to function. However, when we set up the client and his disease (their representatives), it invariably turns out that there is some psychological dynamics between the sick person and his illness.

What does the constellation work on somatic diseases consist in? One could imagine that having a representative of the client and a representative of his illness, we would do some ritual aimed at leaving the disease behind the door. After all, diseases are something we want to get rid of. Hellinger says that when the illness knocks on our door:

> [. . .] instead of opening the door, we try to bolt it, so that it does not come near us and crush us to the ground or confine us to bed. We do not ask what it really is that wants to enter. Thus, we may miss something life-saving that is hidden behind the illness, because we do not want to reach it, despite the fact that it belongs to us and that our heart has secretly waited for its knocking for a long time. (Hellinger 2016, 25–26)[2]

In constellations, we go a different way. We aim at connecting what was separated. Hellinger maintains that the organ in dissonance with us is in resonance with someone else. In this way someone who is excluded manifests himself through the pain and indisposition of our body. The illness is like a reminder of this person. An act of acceptance is therefore obvious, which does not mean that it is easy.

In addition to representing the excluded person, other factors may also play a part in somatic diseases, which is why, as Hellinger says, we must not "reduce the illness to the role of representing an excluded person" (Hellinger 2011, 117). It may result from atonement or following someone into death. In addition, psychological factors not yet discovered, not to mention obvious physical factors, perhaps play a role here.

When the client accepts what manifests itself in the constellation, the representative of the illness immediately feels released and withdraws. In such a case, the forces supporting the illness also disappear. The effects are sometimes spectacular. In my practice, the clients related remission of advanced cancer, recovery from allergy, asthma, persistent back pain, rectal bleeding, cardiac arrhythmia, skin problems, thyroid dysfunction, improvement of the musculoskeletal system, improvement of eyesight, to mention but a few.

I will now address particular diseases. Heart problems, according to Hellinger, are determined by suppressed, unexpressed love. It cannot be surprising that the reason is love, because the heart is undoubtedly related to it—in defiance of cardiology and academic psychology, that want to see it just as a pump. This feeling-related function of the heart can very often be felt directly. When we love someone, we have feelings in the heart area. It is not just that the heart beat gets faster. We can feel what is best called heart opening. In antiquity, the heart was considered to be the source of will, inspiration, and motivation. It is enough that we refer to *The Iliad* or *The Odyssey*, and we will see that the characters described there "think" with their hearts. Lowen writes:

> We all recognize the heart as a symbol of love. But is the relationship between the heart and love only symbolic? Or is there a real and vital connection? Most people have experienced not only a rapid heartbeat in the presence of a loved one but also the heaviness of heart that follows a lovers' quarrel. Moreover, it is common practice in all cultures to place a hand over the heart when talking about love, as if to locate the physical sensations that accompany the emotion. If the heart is involved in every experience of love, as it seems to be, then we must assume that such expressions as a "heart filled with love" also describe a physical phenomenon. (Lowen 2004, 1)

In constellations, the heart additionally seems to be a "transpersonal" organ, it can be "lost" or "given away." It is a kind of energetic "bridge" to another person. Heart problems, for example, arrhythmia, may result from some kind of identification of one's own heart with the heart of someone else, most likely the parent. Our heart begins to "beat to the rhythm of another heart" and problems arise.

Winston was in his fifties and his mother was over 90 years old. Three years earlier, she fainted for cardiological reasons and an ambulance took her. Winston witnessed this and experienced ventricular fibrillation about two hours later (he had not had such serious heart problems before). Winston felt very uncertain in his relationship with the mother, but he was strongly attached to her. Winston's mother humiliated his father, she did not respect him, which caused—normal for a boy—uncertainty whether he was accepted by her. His attachment and uncertainty formed a conglomerate of ambivalent feelings toward the mother. The constellation revealed that Winston was in some sense identified with his mother at the level of the heart—he "gave her his heart." The solution for the client was to accept his mother, stop being afraid of her, and "accept his heart as his own"—which meant letting himself to make his own choices, including emotional ones.

Xenia had a thyroid problem. I set her up in person and a representative of her thyroid. I asked if anyone else in the family had similar problems. It turned out that Xenia's mother had them. I brought in the "mother's thyroid," and then also the "mother." Xenia strongly reacted to the representative of her own thyroid, she cried. After some time both of them sat on the floor and the "thyroid" said that Xenia did not let it protect her, that she took over its functions. The "mother's thyroid" was lying on the floor shielding its head, full of fear, as if it was fighting for life. Soon it became clear to the mother's representative that the "mother's thyroid" was a child. She hugged it, and at that time Xenia's "thyroid" was hugging Xenia. After some time the mother said that the child's father was missing in the constellation, so I brought in his representative. Now everyone was sitting close together on the floor. Then Xenia said with tears, "It's very hard for me to say it, but . . . "—she did not say anything for a long time, she cried. In the end, she started to say, as if to her father, that his deeds had hurt her, that she still remembered being hit on the head. Saying this, she kept looking at the representative of her mother's thyroid (child), although her father was represented by the man who was sitting next to her. I interrupted her: "The father is always an excuse. You are bound to this child and his pain, you are looking at his head, now look consciously. It was the head of that child that was in danger." Xenia felt the bond and cuddled the child. Now she felt calm, and the grievance against her father disappeared at once.

What did this constellation show? The thyroid problems had something to do with Xenia's fearful and constantly defensive attitude. She saw herself as her father's victim, while in reality she identified herself with another victim—a child, perhaps a sibling unknown to her. She could not surrender to the "protection" of her thyroid, just as she distrusted her parents. Only when the forgotten child found his place, could Xenia accept the protection of her thyroid.

Vertigo may be a nonspecific reaction to systemic disorder resulting from family secrets and exclusions. Dyspnea, even lasting for years, can cease as soon as we take into the heart the older brother or sister who died in childhood, which shows that this symptom may also be caused by suppressed love. Nausea may be associated with something "disgusting" that one could not look at, and because of this it became a burden to the descendants. Backache can be a very nagging problem, preventing normal functioning. According to Hellinger, it may be related to an unmaterialized bow. During constellations, it happens that at some moments the representative feels pain in the back, which may be a bodily signal indicating problems with hierarchy and balance, indicating that we take on ourselves something that does not belong to us. Back stiffness may express similar stiffness in one's inner attitude.

Sometimes clients arrive at my office and complain about dysfunctions that surprise me, because they seem purely physical, and even seem to be something too trivial to work on. However, experience has taught me not to underestimate these cases. An example is Mariana's case. She told me about her teenage daughter's problem—she could not put on her contact lenses. It was only during the constellation that Mariana said about her daughter's other fears and resistance related to her body. I stood as Mariana's daughter and put a sheet of paper on the floor representing her problem. Mariana stood next to it. The sheet representing the problem soon began to represent—based on my sensations and conversation with the client—her miscarried child. As Mariana's daughter, I walked around the mother and child, as if they were one extended body. This "body" was sensitive and could not be touched. The daughter identified with its sensitivity. It was a kind of fear of what concerns a woman and her body. I asked the mother to say to her daughter, "This is a woman's life. This is my life. You are a woman too." On the one hand, these words assured the daughter that what belonged to the mother remained with the mother, and on the other—enabled her to accept femininity and her own body. The point was to make the "extended, sensitive body" formed by the mother and the aborted child disappear for the daughter and make her able to identify with her own body.

SYSTEMIC PSYCHO-ONCOLOGY

Simonton and Hellinger

Cancer patients constitute a specific group. They suffer from the disease known as the emperor of all maladies, whose treatment absorbs truly imperial means. They are surrounded by complex equipment and wage a struggle in which surgical operations, radioactive materials, cyclotrons, and very expensive chemical substances are used. A patient who finds himself in the middle of this process will find it difficult to believe that cancer will recede when he changes his mental attitude or takes part in something seemingly as insignificant as a constellation. It is a problem faced by psycho-oncology, whose ambition is to influence the condition of patients. Carl O. Simonton, who developed the first psychotherapeutic system for cancer patients, faced this problem (Simonton et al. 1978, 1992). Although his first patient, a so-called "hopeless case," cured himself through visualization, he did not meet with favor or even with the interest of medical circles. Also, less than half of the patients who were offered Simonton's method, wanted to participate in his program (Wirga 1998, 34). This contradicts the thesis that patients will do anything to recover.

Simonton argued that psychological stress is an important factor in the genesis of cancer, and he focused on helping patients cope with it. This could be achieved by changing too pessimistic beliefs about cancer, creating a greater sense of control over one's own body and pain, strengthening faith in the effectiveness of treatment, improving self-esteem and self-identity, building hope, and emotional honesty. He also pointed to the need to overcome injury and forgiveness. All these elements were supposed to improve the psychophysical state of patients and in this way cause a decrease in the production of anomalous cells and activate the immune system.

Simonton also pointed to the need to identify morbid gains, such as the satisfaction of the need for care, which can be an anchor that keeps us wanting to be sick. He recommended meditation and visualization that were to support the immune system through the influence of imagery on physical processes (e.g., "soldiers"—white blood cells attack the "enemy," i.e., cancer cells).

But that is not all, Simonton acknowledged the importance of the dimension he described as spiritual:

> I believe that, beyond the body and mind, there is another aspect of healing that needs to be addressed: the spiritual aspect. Our work with patients has demonstrated that health involves body, mind and spirit. And while the mind alone can be used to influence the physical state, it is used most effectively when it is aware of spirit. Spirit gives us resources that can't be reached through traditional psychological approaches. It opens us to healing forces that go far beyond our current understanding of our own limits. And we can learn to bring that power into our lives. (Simonton et al. 1992, 13–14)

It resembles Hellinger's words and brings us closer to the systemic understanding of cancer. There is yet another thing. This is what Simonton says about cancer:

> Most people in our culture think that having cancer is terrible luck, a meaningless, random blow of fate. [. . .] But I believe that the message of cancer is always a message of love. (Simonton et al. 1992, 54)

Cancer is not bad luck, it wants to teach us something, and it is a "message of love." Based on the experience provided by constellations, we can understand this surprising thesis, perhaps even better than Simonton himself. Cancer is a result of a deep bond of love with someone from the family system. This bond cries out to be noticed and recognized. In constellations, we put emphasis on the love that flows from us (in accordance with the sentence, that the "move is up to the child") and not the one we are given. A similar conclusion was reached by psychologist David McClelland, who said that the longing and ability to love are more important for our health than how much we are loved by others (Dreher 1996, 213). In constellations, we associate it mainly with the generational system, and we understand it perfectly well—for the health of a child, also with cancer, it is more important to be able to harmoniously express his bond with his mother and other members of the system than their assurance of love. Similarly an adult, if he can love his mother and father without ambivalence and resentment, or realizes his deep bond with one of the ancestors, he will be healthier than a person "surrounded by love."

Like Hellinger, Simonton referred to the forces that go beyond an individual in the exercises for patients:

> Imagine the direction of your path being reinforced by the entire world, the entire universe [. . .]. And now imagine that you understand more of what is going on and has been going on in your life [. . .]. Honor the messages coming in from the whole world; honor the belief that the whole universe wants you to be who you are and will help you be who you are. [. . .] Imagine that the entire world, the entire universe, rejoices because your joy is felt everywhere and your harmony adds to the harmony of the whole world, the whole universe. (Simonton et al. 1992, 83–84)

Systemic constellations give us a better understanding of our past and present life. We also become aware that outside of our ego, there are self-existent forces that are closely connected with us. These forces aim at good, and we are all captured by them. They open before us a deeper and truer image of our place in the world. So one can actually say, "the universe wants us to be who we are and will help us be who we are." We do not learn about it theoretically, but through experiencing the constellation. It becomes clear that cancer is not simply an "enemy that needs to be disposed of," but it does have a function on our path of life. It usually leads us to the people with whom we are connected, and whom we do not remember or rejected on the conscious plane. Speaking even more generally, it leads us to the truth of our lives.

These experiences enhance the sense of connection with wider systems, even with the entire cosmos. Systemic constellations follow the path—pointed also by Simonton—that is not narrowly understood psychology and psychosomatics, but an openness to the spiritual dimension.

This is also evident in Simonton's work on the fear of death and the dying process. He offered his patients a confrontation with the issue of their own death, and those who faced it were able to calm down and even improve their health in the last period of their lives. This corresponds to Hellinger's work with people whose chances of recovery were minimal. Also, Simonton's program contains elements surprisingly similar to what Hellinger suggests to people who want to follow the dead. In such cases, Hellinger suggests that they imagine themselves lying down next to the dead, while Simonton proposes the following visualization:

> See yourself dead. What happens to your consciousness? Let your consciousness go off to wherever you believe your consciousness goes after death. Stay there quietly for a few moments and experience that. (Simonton et al. 1978, 226)

All this is based on a deeply spiritual belief that we will receive from God or the universe what we need, but not necessarily what we want now. This attitude was promoted by Simonton, and his entire system of help closely corresponds to the way of treatment proposed by Hellinger. Simonton names 12 principles of his treatment program (Simonton 2004):

- We are healthy by nature.
- There are ways to increase our vital force, vital energy, and desire to live.
- It is important to effectively resolve emotional distress.
- Imagery is a primary tool in the healing process.
- Hope plays a positive role in the healing process.
- One should not get attached to the outcome (vision of recovery) too much.
- It is important to create healthier beliefs about death and the associated spiritual beliefs.
- One should identify significant patterns of important life events, illness, and the secondary gains of illness.
- One needs to find meaning in the experience of being ill.
- We should explore our intuitive wisdom and basic issues of spirituality.
- It is important to know the principles of support and communication.
- One should create effective life plans.

So the point is to let our body work according to its nature, because it is health-oriented. To believe in the wisdom of the body, which we forget more and more. To increase our inner life energy, we should focus on things that are important to us and give us joy. We must learn to reduce emotional distress, create and maintain our hope and protect it from those who would like to undermine it. At the same time, it is important not to be attached to the outcome, not to stick to the vision of recovery at all costs. This also applies to the person that helps. This recommendation may seem antithetical to the one that says we ought to maintain hope and to the weight that Simonton attaches to the process of imagining positive outcomes of therapy. So how should we understand it? Strenuous sticking to the vision of recovery is blind and may lead to denying the seriousness of the situation. Focusing on a positive result also generates more anxiety and tension. It is difficult, but the work on getting well must integrate acceptance of the possibility of death.

Hellinger very often emphasized the importance of looking death in the eye, and at the same time recognizing its strength. For the sick person, it may be important to calmly look at it and let it give us its message. Then death may withdraw, both in the constellation and reality. Simonton expresses this with the words: "The more we are able to resolve issues of death the more we are able to live life." Simonton also says that our beliefs about death may be healthy or not. It may happen that someone declares that they want to die. What should the therapist do then? Simonton advises to ask the patient: "How do you want to die? What do you think will happen to you after you die?" So the Simonton therapist deals with the topic that is usually considered irrelevant in other forms of therapy. And yet, it is there, "on the other side," that the fantasies that guide us are anchored, which Hellinger showed as the movement toward death and following the dead.

Simonton maintains that one should identify his own patterns of illness and life events. It is difficult to find a tool that would be more useful for this purpose than systemic constellations, in which we discover transgenerational patterns of our fate and diseases. When we set up the patient and his illness, a dynamics immediately arises between them. One can often see that the disease represents a person or leads to some persons. For example, it looks at the dead and also tries to show them to us. Here we move to the next element of the Simonton program, which says that it is very important to express and accept signs of love from the persons close to us and learn to communicate with them, because—as he argues—poor communication with the important people in our lives is one of the biggest stressors. Is communication with the loved ones not the essence of constellations? What is more, constellations make us aware of how many of those significant persons there are. They make it possible for us to feel their love and our love for them. A constellation improves our relationships with the family members (it can also heal our intimate relationships), which gives us a huge boost of energy that is felt directly, and strengthening vital energy is also part of the Simonton therapy.

Another theme that is present throughout the entire Simonton method is the emphasis on strengthening authenticity, being oneself, doing what expresses us, and is not just a habit, pattern, or obligation taken from outside. The point is to be able to say "Yes" and "No." A person struggling with cancer should strengthen in himself what is genuinely his, what belongs to the essence of his personality. I believe there may be something very important here, which, however, has not been accentuated. As we know, the essence of the immune system is the recognition of antigens, "foreign bodies," and then combating them. I think Simonton assumed the seemingly naive belief that being oneself, expressing one's passions, desires, and emotions—so a kind of delineation of a clearer border between "me" and "not-me"—can translate into greater somatic integration. In other words, if I accept who I am and identify with myself, my immune system will also more fully "understand" which cells are "me" and which are not.

If we look at the issue of our psychophysical, and thus also immunological functioning, from this perspective, systemic constellations seem to be a fundamental method in this case too. As we know, systemic entanglements consist in identification with someone from the family. Thus, the border between us and that person gets blurred. We start to live a life that is not ours. Also when we unconsciously want to carry somebody's burden or atone for something that we have not done—then we live somebody else's life. The constellation is a powerful return to oneself, feeling one's borders, both in time (if we interfered in the affairs of the dead) and space (if, for example, we identified with the father or mother). During the constellation, we can also work through guilt and the need for punishment. And Simonton underlines the importance of not feeling guilty.

Let us go further. There is no doubt that constellations confront us with the existence of inner wisdom and intuition. This is already shown by the fact that representatives are able to receive information about completely unknown persons and their problems. So we begin to realize that we are not just biological machines, but part of wider, invisible reality. Such awareness can be very important for a sick person. It makes him sure that there is more happening in his life than psychiatry or oncology knows. Therefore, the patient may be less paralyzed by what is happening around him, which he never fully understands and cannot control. However, he has the resources and the ability to do something within himself and in the accompanying extrasensory reality. Will it not be a huge boost of energy and strength from the regained sense of self-efficacy?

The question arises: Have systemic constellations discovered a kind of psychological (spiritual) causes of cancer? It is difficult to negate the fact that when working with sick people we see very meaningful images. As the heads of the Austrian Society of Psycho-oncology, Hans Peter Bilek and Günther Linemayr, wrote:

> With all restraint, we believe that Bert Hellinger made a significant discovery here, and we would like to justify this by the authenticity with which the protagonists [representatives] communicate their feelings. Authentic perception—both outward and inward—is undoubtedly the main point of psychotherapeutic work and a prerequisite for constructive life changes. From this knowledge, we can also derive a justified hope that in the future Hellinger's way will have an important position in the overall concept of the spiritual treatment of cancer patients. (in: Hellinger 2004, 10)[3]

The "Type C" Personality

Lydia Temoshok developed the concept of "type C" personality, she specified certain character traits that contribute to cancer (Temoshok and Dreher 1992).

She observed that people with this type of personality repress emotions, are excessively polite, and focused on how others perceive them, have a tendency to sacrifice too much to be accepted. Lawrence LeShan also points to hiding behind the façade of gentleness, inability to get angry, lack of spontaneity in contacting other people, dependence on the environment, as well as to feelings of guilt, abandonment and loneliness, shallowness and instability of relationships, lack of satisfaction (LeShan 1994). LeShan argues that such behaviors result from parental rejection or loss, which causes feelings of hurt, abandonment and anxiety, and the belief that close relationships with others bring pain and disappointment. People susceptible to cancer also experience suppressed anger and resentment.

Do systemic constellations confirm the above conclusions? Searching for the causes of cancer in personality traits should be defined as a simplification; however, there is no doubt that there is a connection between the disease and one's mental attitude.

Nadia had lung cancer with metastases to the liver and brain. Yet she always smiled, even when she spoke about difficult matters. Her one-and-a-half-year-old brother drowned before her birth. The constellation showed, among other things, that her mother was unable to mourn his death and to overcome trauma. Nadia said that her mother "often told her how it had happened," but it seemed that those stories—including the one about the postman who did not close the door—were a kind of veil and helped her not face the loss. They certainly burdened Nadia, who felt guilty for many things in her life. She did not consciously blame herself for the death of her brother or her mother's condition, instead, she blamed herself for the abortion she had had. However, during the constellation, the aborted child did not feel that she turned to him with love. Her blaming herself was a barrier for love.

In the course of the constellation, the great-grandmother and some unknown person connected with her were also represented. They were lying next to each other. The great-grandmother's representative felt that a perpetrator and victim were involved, but she did not know whether she was one or the other in this constellation. At one point, the great-grandmother approached the client and said she was her great-grandmother. "Great-granny," Nadia corrected her. "No, great-grandmother," said the representative. She also said that "she was both good and bad." I understood what she meant—Nadia was to take her great-grandmother as she was, not to try to make her turn into "granny." The difficulty with accepting the "great-grandmother" corresponded with Nadia's complaisant way of being.

When the long and complex constellation was coming to an end, I asked Nadia if she now had more energy, if she was more focused on life. She replied, "I always . . . " It was symptomatic—in this way, the client intimated that nothing important had happened.

I understood how strongly Nadia denied and that she did not take her condition seriously. I set up Nadia, her mother and "death." Then I positioned "life" too. Death wanted to dance and play with Nadia, and she, with a fixed smile, pushed it away. In fact, death showed Nadia's nonchalant attitude toward it. Life went out of the room. I asked death and the mother to sit on chairs, and Nadia to stand in front of them. Nadia accepted her mother apparently. But everyone in the group saw her anger. She herself—as before, when she was talking about the partner who had left her with her child—denied it. I said I did not believe what she was saying and encouraged her to contact her emotions. In the end she choked out, "Yes, I'm angry with you. For not fighting, for being weak! I am not like that."

Nadia's mother died of cancer just after her fifties. When she heard the diagnosis, she apparently broke down. Despite her difficult condition, Nadia was optimistic. That optimism was nothing but a turning away from the gravity of the situation. She had to radiate it to show her mother that she was different, better. When Nadia acknowledged her negative feelings for the mother, the representative of life spontaneously came closer (which is a typical reaction in the moments when emotional truth appears).

Finally, I again asked Nadia to accept the mother. She said she was accepting her and waiting for them to meet again. Nadia was a Jehovah's Witness and emphasized that such a meeting was obvious to her. I intuitively asked, "That's a stupid question, but why do you want to meet your mother?" Nadia: "To embrace her. And to say that I didn't break down, that I fought . . . " At that moment, many people within the group sighed, and I interrupted Nadia. It was a continuation of her exaltation above the mother and accusing her. I said emphatically and sharply that if she did not change her attitude, life would soon show her how much her fight meant. That it would prove that she was just like her mother.

Nadia's case is an example of repression of anger, an attempt to be only good (which was further strengthened by the ethos of Jehovah's Witnesses) and the destructive function of false optimism, which ultimately caused her to go toward death with a smile and nonchalance. My client reminds one of Temoshok's patients, about whom she writes:

> Elizabeth seemed to believe that the only way to stay strong and positive was to erase negative feelings from her mind and heart. [. . .] With the support of her family and her religious faith, Elizabeth was untouched by fear. "I face the fear with faith," she told me. She repeated these words like a mantra throughout our interview. [. . .] She'd lived her life to give care, and saw her illness as another opportunity to reach out to people in need. "Maybe this is a way for me to be even more compassionate in my work with Alzheimer's patients," she said. (Temoshok and Dreher 1992, 31)

Leo also demonstrated the attitude of denying negative emotions. When he stood in front of the mother's representative, he said with a smile, "Yes, of course I accept her. Mother is such a woman that can't be unaccepted." However, neither me nor the mother's representative felt that those were his true feelings. Like his father, he also had some resistance and shyness toward his mother. Leo gave the impression of a dovish person, having harmonious relationships with his family and the world. But I do not think that this attitude was mature and achieved consciously. It was rather a group of infantile defense mechanisms. This situation resulted from the interrupted movement of love that we worked on in the further part of the constellation.

Hellinger said that it is easy to tell who of those with cancer will live and who will die—those who are afraid of death belong to the first group. Temoshok confirms this seemingly surprising statement:

> Many patients told me they weren't the least bit anxious about having cancer. They used the defense of denial to completely block awareness of fear. These were individuals who could not tolerate fear, and my impression was that they'd been that way since childhood. Morton, a forty-year-old maintenance man, lived alone with his mother and sister. He told me that finding out he had cancer "didn't bother me, didn't faze me." He added, "I don't really think I have cancer anymore." The only thing about cancer that made him anxious, he said, was the big-city traffic he would hit on his way into San Francisco for doctor's appointments. (Temoshok and Dreher 1992, 35)

Cancer and Mother

There are many types of cancer. However, breast and genital organ tumors in women are often conditioned by their attitude toward the mother or the nature of the relationships in their maternal line. Bert Hellinger argued:

> Women suffer from cancer when their mothers have no place in their hearts. Then illness can be atonement for this injustice. (Hellinger and Nehrebecki 2012, 58)[4]

This may be a multigenerational pattern: a woman with cancer rejects her mother, who held a grudge against her mother, who did not accept her own mother. The sick woman can exalt herself above the mother, and if she has children—consider herself to be better as a mother. She may reject her mother when the mother is emotionally unavailable due to her being tied to someone else, for example, her deceased siblings. Rejection of the mother often results in understating the weight of motherhood, aversion to having children and fertility issues.

Health in such cases returns primarily through the acceptance of the mother and this what comes from the female line of ancestors. This requires respect for the hierarchy and recognition that the woman has received everything that is female, namely fertility and reproductive organs, from her mother. Hellinger says that "no one can be healthy without a bond with the mother" (Hellinger and Nehrebecki 2012, 57).[5]

The more the daughter gets used to the undue position in the family, the more difficult it is for her to accept the mother. One of my cancer patients, Agnes, stressed that her "father loved her more than he loved her mother." During the constellation her representative felt lofty and tried to control her mother's behavior.

Tamara suffered from endometriosis for many years, and for some time also from a strange—as she called it—type of cancer, because the tumors "wandered" around the ovaries, fallopian tubes, and uterus. The doctors insisted on cutting out the internal reproductive organs, but Tamara did not submit to an operation. The constellation revealed that Tamara's great-grandmother had some traumatic experiences possibly related to her children. Tamara knew there was a conflict between her mother and grandmother, and it was manifested in the constellation. Tamara herself often complained about her mother, she considered her to be cold and indifferent. The constellation revealed that Tamara's mother was inwardly focused on the trauma of the great-grandmother.

The solution for Tamara was a movement toward her mother, which was possible only after she realized why her mother had isolated herself. Only then could she understand that not everything in her life was the mother's fault. Her parents moved abroad when Tamara was four years old, which made her feel that there was a break in the continuity of her life (for example, she forgot her mother tongue). Now, however, she could look at it as part of her fate, from which one can also derive strength.

Alina was diagnosed with a tumor in mediastinum about a month before the constellation. She had a difficult relationship with her mother and in her childhood she did not feel attached to her. When she was nine years old, the mother moved out with Alina's newborn half-brother, and she stayed with her mother's parents. She did not have contact with her father either, despite the fact that he lived nearby. She said that she would like her mother to understand how important the family is, that everyone should meet together. But the mother was "rejecting and thick-skinned."

The constellation revealed Alina's need for control. Her representative wanted to order the whole family around and show her mother what was right. Alina, despite the external attitude of openness and declaration of the desire to reconcile, internally despised her mother, considering herself to be better. It manifested itself, for example, in this seemingly positive sentence:

"My children fare better, because it fared so badly with me." When I added a representative of her cancer, there was an immediate attraction between Alina and "cancer," they both smiled happily at each other. The "tumor" gave Alina strength. She needed it to order around the family and be better than her mother.

It was characteristic that when Alina's representative took an internal step toward recognizing her own limitations, that is, toward being the mother's child and taking her place in the system, "cancer" felt that it could move away. However, it was difficult for Alina to let it go forever. She could not accept her mother and her position as a child. When she stood at a certain distance from her mother and could not get close, I positioned "cancer" between them with its arms outstretched in their direction as if it were joining them. It suited Alina, but it did not suit the mother. After that intervention, Alina explained that shortly before her illness she had imagined that she had been dying and that everyone would unite at her funeral. Thus, death or cancer would give her special power to take a meta-systemic position, that is, to be more than just a child and control the situation. The cure was a change in that mental attitude—abandoning the omnipotent aspirations, taking her place in the system and accepting the mother as a mother.

Eleanor, fifty years old, had a surgery to remove her uterus, ovaries, and fallopian tubes and some lymph nodes due to cancer over a year before the constellation. Soon after the surgery, it turned out that a new tumor appeared in the peritoneum. During the initial interview, I learned that Eleanor's father was dead; two grandmother's sisters committed suicide (one of them probably suffered from postpartum depression and jumped out of the window); two brothers of the mother died tragically (one in a mine, the other was hit by a tram). Eleanor has two sons, one from the first marriage.

I set up Eleanor and a representative of "cancer or what was behind it." The client sat down, and after a while, the representative of cancer sat down too, with the words: "I will also sit down because I don't want to have power over you." After a while she said, "There's only one thing in my head: first husband." Since I had already been attracted to this field, I lay down between Eleanor and the representative of cancer. I began to spontaneously stretch my arms toward both persons, as if I wanted to connect them somehow. I asked the client what had happened to her first husband. She said he was dead but could not tell me anything more. I replied that, of course, if she did not want to, she did not have to, but suggested that she think about it again and perhaps she would be able to tell something.

As an afterthought, Eleanor said, "OK, I'll say it, I aborted my pregnancy." I positioned the aborted child. The tumor said it wanted to leave and did not want to "torment" her, to which Eleanor replied, "What you want doesn't matter." The work consisted in admitting the loss and responsibility for what had happened to the child. Eleanor said she felt ashamed of the abortion, but the shame was a form of resistance to a real confrontation with the loss and responsibility. She tried to hug the child, but it moved away from her, sensing the lack of acceptance. The "tumor" represented what was real and emotional in her. Saying that "cancer" was part of herself, I asked the client to say to it: "I accept you."

The constellation revealed the conflictual relationship with the mother—it was difficult for Eleanor to look at her, she reproached her. She said that the mother had been constantly looking after her younger, severely burned in childhood, brother. When the brother lay down next to the mother, Eleanor said, "That's how it's always been." The client, displaying enormous jealousy of her brother, said with a grudge to her mother's representative, "I don't exist." She meant that she was not important, that to her mind she did not exist to her mother. However, in her situation these words expressed something much more important—her own withdrawal from life.

After the constellation, I did a simple exercise with all the participants of the therapeutic group: standing in a circle, we held our hands, and I suggested that we let everything we had blocked flow through our hands, from the left to the right and vice versa. It was supposed to be both what we considered to be bad and what we thought was good. At the end, I asked if anyone had difficulty doing the exercise or if someone did not feel the flow. Eleanor said she was stiff from the navel to the neck, she felt nothing. I asked her to lie down on a blanket. I put a hand on her chest, I asked her how she felt—she replied that it was the warmth of my hand. I asked, what came to her mind, what words, images:

E: Emptiness—this word comes to my mind.
T: When did this emptiness appear in your life? When did it come to you?
E: I don't know . . . When I was one year old.
T: What happened then?
E: Mom left me at my grandma's.

I asked the person who had previously represented Eleanor's mother to sit down beside her and put a hand on her chest. Eleanor said she felt as if she had had a "brick" there. It was clear that it was due to the interrupted movement of love toward the mother and isolation from her.

Maya, a woman in her early forties, had tumors in various parts of the body. The client had a sister, a year and a half older than her, and the mother supposedly did not expect to get pregnant a second time—"if she realized earlier that she was pregnant, she would have probably terminated the pregnancy." Maya said that she actually wanted to die. She said that she was not afraid of death because she knew that "it was fine, wonderful there." However, she had a son and wanted to live for him. When I listened to her, I felt that what she was saying did not sound serious. Later in the conversation, Maya said, "I *killed* two loves" and "Mother *killed* that love"—in both cases, she meant her ex-boyfriends.

At the beginning of the constellation, I laid a representative of Maya down suggesting that she was an infant, and the representative of her older sister beside her. I also positioned the mother's representative. The mother said that "the child's [Maya's] attitude towards the world annoyed her" and that she had a bond with Maya's sister, but it was difficult for her to have a close relationship with Maya. Guided by the systemic intuition, I laid "someone earlier" behind Maya, and after a while, one more person (perhaps even earlier). After some time, I asked Maya and her sister to stand up. I positioned "death." Maya's representative moved away from "death," and the sister shielded Maya, facing "death." Maya said to it, "Go away, you're not needed here."

I asked Maya herself to enter the constellation, stand next to the sister and mother. She felt a great weakness, began to close her eyes, staggered (the representatives had to support her), she did not want to look at "death." I said, "Don't flee from death into death." Finally, Maya could look at it. I asked her to say to it, "I've been always afraid of you. So much." I turned Maya around and led her "towards life"—showing the view outside the window (it is a good representation of life). Maya said, "Life's not so nice at all." I turned her around again. Holding her by the shoulders and shaking her slightly, I said that I thought she was a small child who imagined that she was big, bigger than life, bigger than the universe (this is how I conceptualized her mental attitude, standing next to her and tuning into her field). Behind the mother, I positioned the client's grandmother, then the grandmother's mother (great-grandmother) and her mother (great-great-grandmother). Maya approached her grandmother and hugged her tightly. Then the mother said she loved her. Maya stood at a distance, looked at the mother and cried, she asked her to once again say that she loved her. The process of accepting the mother started.

This constellation suggests how omnipotent and self-destructive the fantasies of a child who feels cut off from the mother can be. Maya had to experience great fear of being abandoned and of death, and to deal with it, she created a sense of nonchalance in relation to life and death. To some extent, she needed a life-threatening illness to prove herself that she had no fears. Her story of believing in an afterlife was not mature—it stemmed from her infantile thinking and overwhelming fear.

Something similar took place, when I worked with a cancer patient, Doris. She told me that when she was examined a few years ago and heard she was healthy, she felt sad. At some point in the constellation, with tears and great pain, she said to her mother's representative, "Mom, let me die, it'll be better this way." It was shocking. I asked, "Why do you hate your mother so much?" The client was unable to answer or accept the mother and her own life. I stood as her "resistance," the cause of that inability. I straightened up, lifted my head high and walked, "high and mighty," in front of the group. There was some kind of bizarre loftiness in it. But where did it come from? I did not blame the client, that pride—probably of a child—must have had a root. The further course of the constellation showed that that pride was a defense against anxiety (which probably resulted from the identification with the child aborted by the mother and at the same time from the reluctance to look at him as a child). Here too, omnipotence had a defensive dimension.

A Tumor Representing the Fetus?

For a long time, cancer development was seen as a gradual accumulation of random mutations, which was in agreement with the mechanistic approach of science. In this view, cancer is simply a chaotic tumor. However, Isaac S. Kohane's research shows that cancer is something much more organized:

> Analyzing tumors from dozens of tissue types, Isaac S. Kohane of the Harvard-MIT Division of Health Sciences and Technology has catalogued surprising yet familiar patterns of gene activity in cancer cells—they are the same programmed genetic instructions active during various stages of embryonic and fetal development. Entire suites of genes that drive an embryo's early growth and the later formation of limbs and other structures in the womb normally go silent during the rest of life, but these genetic programs are switched back on in many tumor cells. (Soares 2009)

A pioneering researcher on cancer, Lloyd J. Old, maintains that the concept that cancer and development are related originated long ago, as in the nineteenth century pathologist John Beard noticed similarities between tumors and the trophoblast, a part of an early embryo from which the placenta is formed at a later stage. Old said that "'the trophoblast invading the uterus [. . .] invades, spreads, creates a blood supply. It also suppresses the maternal immune system,'" which is "'characteristics of cancer.'" The researcher identified genetic programs common to tumor cells and gametes and called cancer a "somatic cell pregnancy" (Soares 2009).

Physicist Paul Davies, together with his colleagues, developed the "atavistic theory of cancer," according to which cancer is understood as the result of very ancient genetic programs. The author writes:

> Metastasis—the process whereby normally sedentary cells become mobile, quitting a tumour to spread around the body—mimics what happens during early-stage embryogenesis, when immature cells are often not anchored in place but surge in organized patterns to designated locations. (Davies 2019, 136)

How does this correspond to systemic constellations? First of all, in constellations, we recognize the "meaning of the disease," that is, cancer does not only result from random and mechanical mutations. Second, if tumor activates embryonic programs, that is, it is somewhat similar to an embryo, then it coincides with our vision of cancer as a representative of a person. A "somatic cell pregnancy" would be an attempt to revive someone who was excluded in one's own body. Perhaps this is often related to a twin lost during the fetal life. Alfred and Bettina Austermann advanced an identical hypothesis that "the body produces [cancerous] tissue in order to at least have an 'illusory twin' since the true one is not there any more" (Austermann and Austermann 2019, 89). Similarly, Annette Proksch, gynecologist, believes that "the psyche or rather the strong longing for the lost twin can animate the ovaries to form dermoid cysts" (Austermann and Austermann 2019, 65). Some observations lead me to presume that particularly brain cancers in children may result from the prenatal loss of twin siblings. The Austermanns also presume this:

> In connection with the loss of a twin we have worked with several adults and children who had or still have a brain tumor. In some cases it became apparent that the tumor was clearly linked to the prenatal experience of having lost the beloved twin. To some extent the tumor was supposed to replace the closeness to the twin or rather to fill the emptiness that had been left after the other's death. The tumor seemed to be a desperate expression of the big love for the other one. (Austermann and Austermann 2019, 89)

Many people, especially children—as the mechanisms that drive them to death are not so fixed—could be helped if these processes were taken into account by physicians.

NOTES

1. Quotation translated from Polish.
2. Quotation translated from Polish.
3. Quotation translated from German.
4. Quotation translated from Polish.
5. Quotation translated from Polish.

Chapter 10

The Systemic Background of Professional and Business Problems

SYSTEMIC COACHING

Systemic Constellations in Coaching

Coaching is a field of knowledge and practice, whose aim is to help people improve their activities, achieve goals, and implement professional plans, such as becoming effective leaders. Systemic coaching is the application of knowledge and techniques of systemic constellations in coaching, which is possible thanks to the fact that the laws of family systems have proved to be useful also for systems related to work, career, business, and functioning of organizations.

What is the difference between systemic coaching and traditional coaching? Systemic coaching departs from focusing on individuality and perceives each person as part of a larger invisible reality. Hellinger refers to it as "what is," meaning that although externally we may seem to be completely free and undetermined, each of us "carries" a system that affects him. This invisible reality can strengthen our endeavors or impede them. By reaching this sphere of our lives, systemic coaching makes it possible for us to solve issues that are difficult to solve with the use of other methods, and the effects are achieved very quickly.

Jenny Rogers, a coaching theoretician and practitioner, lists a few basic principles of classic coaching (Rogers 2012, 7–8):

- The client has the resources to resolve his problems;
- The coach asks, "the penetrating questions which take clients into territory they have never previously considered";
- The coach does not give advice;

- Coaching addresses the person's past and present experiences, as well as his future, it concerns both his work and private life;
- The client's agenda is important, the coach withdraws his own ideas if they are not consistent with what the client wants to work on;
- The coach and the client are equals, the rule is to suspend judgment and respect each other;
- Coaching is about change and action.

These principles do not conflict with what systemic coaching proposes. Here too we are aware of the client's resources; we are focused on change; we do not judge; and we do not give advice and have respect for the client. We lead him into completely new areas of solutions, which he has definitely not considered before.

There are, however, important differences between classic coaching and systemic coaching. Traditional coaching is based on asking questions that are supposed to lead the client to discover new knowledge. This knowledge is hidden in his mind, more or less deeply, sometimes we say it is in the subconscious.

In systemic coaching, we reach the subconscious knowledge, but we also discover the knowledge that exists outside the client's mind. We derive information from the system in which the client functions. This system—whether it consists of goals, colleagues, or the departments of the enterprise—has its own dynamics. That is why we depart from what the client defines himself toward something more objective, remaining attentive to his goals and needs. Systemic coach John Whittington wrote:

> System dynamics don't respond to assessments of personality type, objective-setting or a new strategic plan. Systems are not affected by the team profile or whether there's a particular conflict model being applied. System dynamics are beyond rational intervention and require something else. They need to be addressed by systemic interventions. (Whittington 2016, 8)

He thinks that classic coaching supports the nonsystemic perspective—the belief that one person or team is strong enough to achieve all their goals. However, "systemic leadership needs to be alert to the energies across the whole system, working in service of the purpose and coherence of the whole system," and not just focus on the individuals and their objectives (Whittington 2016, 12). Leaders generally think that having a clear goal, intention, mission, and tools is the basis for success. But it may turn out to be not enough and the system resists, because "the purpose or the human dynamics around it are not aligned with the systemic organizing forces" (Whittington 2016, 13).

Systemic coaching stems from family work, because the family system is always the basic system for everyone. Business advisor Friedrich Assländer writes that problems in the family system that are unresolved "are often unconsciously externalized in the enterprise" (Grün and Assländer 2009, 119).[1] The author instances a case of two brothers who ran a company together but, despite their attempts to cooperate harmoniously, felt a tension. They were asked to set up their relationship in space:

> The older one stood in the center, put his hands on the hips. The younger one did not find a good place, in the end he stood about two meters away from his brother and explained that this was not a good place, but it was the least worst of all the ones he tried. These places correspond to their proper order in the shared family system. The older one stands before the younger one in accordance to chronology. He appeared in the world first and therefore always puts himself before his younger brother. The reason for the unexplained tensions between the brothers comes to light when they are asked questions about the company's history. The younger of them established the company many years ago, and his older brother joined a few years later. After this explanation, both brothers were asked to switch places. Immediately, a clear change in body posture and facial expression could be observed in both brothers. The older one said that a weight had been lifted off his shoulders. The younger one thought that he had finally found the right place. (Grün and Assländer 2009, 120)[2]

The above example—that illustrates a mingling of two hierarchies: related to the family and to the company—demonstrates the simplicity in reaching important conclusions, characteristic of constellations. It was enough for the brothers to stand with the intention to demonstrate their relationship, and everything began to become clear.

Constellation work shows that we live in a broad context. We often do not notice it or try to bypass it. We then concentrate all our efforts on goals and tasks, but we cannot achieve much. Initially, the constellation we want to work on may involve elements such as the company, business partner, clients, money, headquarters, and new premises. They may seem to be the only significant factors in the reorganization of the company. However, the constellation may show that some other element that has not been considered before, for example, an earlier partner or someone from the client's family, also plays an important systemic role. What seemed unrelated becomes part of the case. An attempt to achieve the goal in an isolated context is doomed to failure. One has to go beyond the hitherto narrow perspective and sometimes confront the past or the denied present state. That is why systemic coaching not only makes better results in business possible, but it is also an avenue for personal growth.

Constellations of Companies and Organizations

Systemic constellations make it possible to work in a wide range of areas, including the company's structure, marketing, financial, and personnel issues. In this context, we refer to constellations of organizations. These constellations enable the organization to function harmoniously and achieve its goals. This only works if the systemic orders are respected, essentially the same orders as in the family system.

This may come as a surprise. There are, after all, many organizations, such as some corporations that violate the systemic orders and yet seem to function well. These organizations lack harmony, there is envy in them, the employees are treated unfairly, and the management is dishonest. How is it possible that they are successful?

If we look at them closer, it will turn out that their successes are superficial and come at a cost of losses. Such successes cost people their health, well-being, and their families also pay the price. Many of these systems function in a state of constant tension and struggle, and new employees feel exploited not only because of a given organizational culture but also for hidden systemic reasons—as a result of the system's striving for balance even at their expense.

Organizational and business constellations:

- Enable to solve difficulties in managing the company and people;
- Show the causes of conflicts in the workplace;
- Make it possible to discover the reasons for the decrease in employee motivation;
- Support structural and personnel changes;
- Help to activate customers' interest in the product or service;
- Uncover the causes of the company's financial problems;
- Eliminate the difficulties in communication and information flow in the enterprise;
- Help to negotiate;
- Enable to find the right place for a given employee in the company.

Many businesses fail, and many companies go bankrupt. It can be assumed that very often systemic factors play a decisive role in these failures. Why do companies fail? There may be many reasons, but lack of customers is one of the most important ones. It is customers who guarantee the survival of any company. Constellations show something very important here. It turns out that customers already have a given attitude toward the company or the product, even when in reality the company has not had a single customer yet! However, these potential customers—along with the company and other key elements—already form a certain virtual, but affecting reality, system. Taking them into account is crucial for the success of the venture.

In a constellation, we can see the root of the lack of clients or their sufficient number. By bringing about the orders, customers get closer to the company in the constellation, which is not limited to a symbol, but has real effects. Let the following case illustrate, how powerful such a constellation can be.

Chloe was responsible for sales in a Polish engineering company, whose product is still a technological novelty, and therefore, the company must prove its advantage over the old methods. This company is a subsidiary of a company based in Scandinavia. In the constellation, markers were used to represent the client, her company, the mother company, product, and customers. A constellation is a multifactorial, dynamic process, where a change in one element entails a change in others, so a causal interpretation of the type: "due to element A, element B . . ." does not always make sense. To simplify, however, we can conclude that the customers kept their distance from the product because of the parent company. It looked as if they were afraid of it. It seems that, among other things, different styles of doing business in Poland and Scandinavia were involved. After the systemic orders were brought about (probably the most important thing was to simply give space to this dynamics in this case), the customers became clearly interested in the product.

A potential customer according to the traditional approach is someone that may be interested in our offer, but he is not interested in it yet. So it seems logical that these people cannot play a real role in the situation of the company. There is no relationship between them and the company yet. Also the company's real customers did not know about its international connections, and all the more did not feel any psychologically understood "fear" of the parent company. And yet the usual logic fails here. In constellations, it is possible to represent potential customers as if they were a real group. It is also possible to change the "attitude" of this group toward the company.

It is indeed a different paradigm and because of its unusual nature it would not have much to say in its defense if it were not for one powerful argument—it works. A few months after the company was set up, inquiries and purchase orders literally started to pour in. The manager related that she was asked twice about the sudden increase in the number of purchase orders: "What's going on?" "But what exactly happened, do you understand it?"

Coaching or Psychotherapy?

Systemic coaching has its roots in family constellations, that is, in therapeutic work. So the question can be asked: Is it not too "deep"? On the other hand, we all have bigger or smaller psychological problems. Thus, a challenge arises for the coaches who rather wish to work with people with a generally "undisturbed" psyche. It happens that the coaching process reaches an impasse or fails due to "deeper" problems in the coachee. It may also be so—I remember such a case from systemic supervision—that coaching becomes for a given person an attempt to cut himself off from what he should first of all deal with. In such a case, the coach works on the surface, unaware of the fact that the client's most difficult issues are hidden from him. In fact, both the coach and the coachee play a game with each other.

A very useful feature of systemic constellations is that we can "dose" the depth of this work and the systemic coach should be able to adjust his work to the requirements and capabilities of the client. We can even work without knowing who or what the individual elements of the system represented are (these are the so-called "covered constellations"). In a given constellation, instead of positioning the "mother," we can set up "something that matters here," and avoid, at least at the first meeting, broaching family issues. On the other hand, the coach working with systemic constellations must be aware of the fact that a considerable part of the client's problems is related to his family system. Therefore, although he does not do this automatically and does not insist on it, he is ready to go with the client in this direction. Whittington says that, taking into account the context and the permission obtained, it is worth sharing with the client the two truths that are obvious in terms of constellations:

- All you need from your parents is life. They've already given you that.
- If you can't receive life from your parents, you will have difficulty resourcing yourself to lead others. (Whittington 2016, 262)

These matters are so unequivocal that it is impossible and pointless to "protect" the client from seeing them. Thanks to systemic constellations, we know very well that there are rules from which there is no deviation. Of course, like all rules, these can also be broken, but this always involves a price to pay. By working with systemic coaching, we do not become psychotherapists, but we are open to the deeper area of the client's psyche that is related to emotions and feelings. Another thing is that, and this is the knowledge based on experience, people turn out to be much more ready to go deeper than we generally think. This happens when they feel that they follow their own process, not something imposed from outside.

When we work as a coach, we often face a situation where relationships deeper than the level at which the client suggested to work reveal themselves. A young man, Raphael, came to a session to work on his university choice. In the constellation, we used the tetralemma. Raphael had actually already applied to one school, but he still wanted to see "what it would be like" and consider the other school. He stood next to the representative of the other school and said that "he felt good and calm here, but he did not know what he was supposed to do here." The school he chose attracted him as if he had a job to do there. It soon became clear that the school he chose represented his mother and the other one—his father.

Raphael was raised only by his mother, who did not have a good opinion of his father (the representative of "both," in this case the parental relationship, felt very bad). He internally submitted to his mother, which was reflected by his choice of school. He lacked something, however, and this made him think about another school. In the constellation, he had a grievance and was angry with his father, but he finally reconciled with him and felt strengthened. Accepting the father made it possible for him to be separated from his mother's desires and point of view, which became the real goal of this constellation. Matthias Varga and Insa Sparrer also speak of the fact that the constellation can represent different levels and smoothly go from testing choices to the family level (Varga and Sparrer 2018, 100).

Of course, coaching work does not always concern the mother and father. Often, it is about the systemic laws, which concern various elements, and which must be taken into account. Sometimes it can be quite simple. Adriana, psychologist, wanted to do something in addition to individual psychotherapy and training. She had a few ideas, for example, manufacturing, but she could not seriously start to implement these ideas. However, she could not explain why. Maybe because she would have less time for the family? Because of the fear of having "something for herself"? Or maybe because of her father, who was always "exhausted" and she expected it should be hard for her too? I asked her to put three pieces of paper on the floor: "individual therapy," "training courses," and "new job." I stood on one of them myself and two other workshop participants stood on the remaining ones. After some time, we all three stood in a row, like siblings, in the following order: "individual therapy," "training courses," "new job." It became clear that the solution was to accept the hierarchy. The client needed to look at it this way: "The therapy is first, then the training courses, and when she finds time, the new activity." It seems very simple, even trivial, but it was concrete information that helped her understand what had seemed very chaotic to her up to that point.

Coaching of the Coach

Constellations not only make it possible to work directly with organizations but also to supervise this kind of work. As in constellations, it can lead to completely unexpected insights. These insights can concern not only the problem brought to supervision by the coach but also the deeper spheres of the personality of the coach himself.

Laura, who is business psychologist and systemic coach, was hired as an external consultant in a fairly large, rapidly growing technology company. However, it was not clear to her what her role actually was. She also suspected that she might be used as someone onto whom the responsibility for firing some employees could be shifted.

I used the technique of chair arrangement. I asked Laura to set up the chairs for the people she spoke about: for herself, for the company owner, for his daughter, who was in charge of the company's finances and was in fact his right hand, although the co-owners and employees were not aware of this. The head of the company often consulted Laura over the phone on various business and interpersonal matters. Laura's representative was sitting next to the owner's representative, and his daughter's representative was sitting opposite them. Laura's representative (hereafter: Laura) immediately felt that she wanted to do her job, she wanted to prove herself competent, and do something significant for the company. The company owner was interested in his daughter, whom he saw, in a somewhat dehumanized way, as if she had been part of the company.

The constellation was complex and multithreaded, so I will focus on what was most important here. Behind Laura, I set up "what she brought into this job." The representative of this element began talking about associations with drugs, alcohol, then a sense of rolling in the mud, and primitive physiological behavior. Laura said with a smile that alcohol and drugs were not alien to her, but that was a long time ago. Later in the constellation, she told us that she had sometimes brought her drunk father, a successful businessman and president of a company, home. It was very humiliating for her.

The constellation revealed her father's conflict, taken over by his daughter, who was closely attached to him. The father came from a poor peasant family and was the only one that went that far. His representative's feelings showed his ambivalence—his escape and, at the same time, his unappeasable longing for the land and something simple, almost physiological. Laura remembered how ashamed she had been and how much she had sympathized with him when his relatives had appeared at some family celebration—extremely simple people, worn out by hard work and living conditions. Both the father and his daughter internally and externally ran away from those roots and were attached to them at the same time. Alcohol and narcotics, as the representatives felt, made it possible to come into contact with that world which was associated with primitivism and physiology.

How did this relate to the client's initial question about her role in the company? Laura understood that she tried to impress the owner of the company and save him as she had done with her father. She gained the opportunity to leave the father's dilemmas and difficulties with him, which opened her up to a more realistic approach to her work. At the end of the constellation, it was also clear that this was a family business—there was the father, the daughter, and, as it turned out, also the son employed there—which was doing well anyway. All this enabled Laura to adopt a calm and balanced attitude toward her tasks.

FAMILY AND SUCCESS

Mother and Father and Success

Bert Hellinger associates the issue of success with the fundamental events in our lives. What is the first success? Our birth. Hellinger writes:

> This is when we had to first prove our ability to assert ourselves. This success continues to work throughout our lives. From this experience, we gain the strength to successfully assert ourselves also later on. (Hellinger 2011a, 10)[3]

Sometimes, subconsciously, we do not believe that this success has really happened. This is a very concrete psychological phenomenon that I discovered while practicing constellations and defined as "incomplete birth." When this kind of problem occurs, the individual lives with only "one foot" in the world, feels as if he does not believe that he has been born, that he has succeeded. This inner attitude is unconscious, but has far-reaching consequences. The individual does not have all the potential life energy, is susceptible to depression, apathy, lack of motivation, and satisfaction with life.

Our second success is accepting the mother. "Every success has the face of the mother," Hellinger says. This is the basic statement regarding the connection between professional success and relationship with our parents. The move toward the mother and taking from her is something active. We must call her and actively suck. The mother is the first person who gives us. Because the mother is the one from whom we learn to take, the blocked path to her leads to inability to take in general. Of course, we still want to get this or that from life, but at a deeper level we cannot take. We think: "I don't want anything, I don't need anything, I'll be self-sufficient." We do not achieve success because we try to persevere with the illusion of self-sufficiency.

It happens that someone actively rejects the mother and internally turns away from her. In this way, they turn away from what is life-giving, causing growth and well-being. When someone rejects their mother, they "reject their life, their work and their profession" (Hellinger 2011a, 11).[4] The mother is the foundation of all success, the starting point. To want success, to be able to take one's success and use it, one has to take the mother into the heart. Freud noticed some of this, because he said:

> If a man has been his mother's undisputed darling he retains throughout life the triumphant feeling, the confidence in success, which not seldom brings actual success along with it. And Goethe might well have given some such heading to his autobiography as: "My strength has its roots in my relation to my mother." (Freud 1955, 156)

Freud does not draw any distinction, but note that he refers to Goethe's relation to his mother and not his mother's relation to him: "My strength has its roots in my relation to my mother." You do not have to be your mother's darling, and the relations with her can be various. In constellations, such or other manifestations of the relationship with the mother are not important, nor is her attitude toward the child. What is important is the child's attitude toward her. And more specifically—taking the mother as a mother. It is difficult for many people. Even if the relationship with the mother is good, the mother may not be fully accepted. This means that someone holds a grudge, blames her, and has persistent, sometimes unconscious infantile expectations toward her. Being in this state, they undermine their creative powers and their own ability to act.

Adele was involved in many activities that did not satisfy her; they were not what she wanted to do. She wanted to go into psychotherapy, but organized so-called "hard skills trainings." In a constellation (with the use of plastic markers), she closed herself in a circle formed by psychotherapy, its clients and the representation of one more activity. By contrast, she moved away from money, trainings, and their clients. So I added a marker defined as "something that is related to her attitude to money." It soon became clear that the added element represented the mother. The client wanted to throw her off the table with everything that stood next to her. She explained that the mother's attitude to money was a burden for her—her mother feared for money, she was often afraid of losing it. Therefore, next to the mother, I set up a representation of "something from the past, that affected the mother's attitude towards money." Perhaps it was related to the great-grandfather, who—as the client said—"had lost everything."

I asked Adele to say internally that she was accepting her mother and leaving everything related to her attitude to money. Then Adele felt that it was hard for her to leave her mother alone with it. For it is easier to reject a mother than to leave her in "trouble." That is why I put "support" for the mother, who was strongly bound to "something from the past," in which the daughter was not allowed to intervene. When Adele felt that these things did not concern her at all, the issues from before she was born, it was easier for her to abandon her destructive loyalty. She gained the opportunity to accept her mother and leave her attitude towards finances with her.

Leaving "mother's money" with the mother or "father's money" with the father and taking "one's own money" is an important process that I have tested in many constellations. It does not always have to be money. Separating "one's own" from that "of the parent" may concern, for example, work or even sex. The point is that the child is, as it were, incapacitated by the parent's projections, opinions, and words, and behaves as if what he does (work, sex, earning money) was not his own. Separating one from the other and regaining certain spheres of life for oneself can never involve rejection of the parent, but always goes through the process of accepting him more fully.

The third pillar of success is the father. We can say that accepting the mother makes us ready to succeed, and accepting the father makes us capable of achieving the success. The father figure is connected with our going to the world, with the ability to adopt social roles and undertake professional activities. The father is the professional life. However, in many companies and institutions, one can feel a deficit of the father. And where there is no internalized father, there are completely inadequate, in professional situations, sulks, lack of borders, blurred competences, lack of authority or respect, and unpunctuality. Superiors who have an internal problem with their father are exposed to constant hesitation, they may be too lenient or the opposite—mindlessly oppressive. Subordinates who have not accepted their father tend to bring their family affairs to work, sometimes they are demanding, and they cannot properly assess the relation of their contribution to remuneration. In such companies, mobbing can also prevail.

What we call masculine energy, the father's energy, is in a particular way important for a man. According to the orders of love, a man should "stand by his father," which means a certain form of acceptance and identification with the male line of the family. This enables him to better realize his potential, which—regardless of various preferences—remains essentially masculine. For this reason, among other things, many homosexual men, who sometimes stand closer to their mother than their father, must give up more masculine professions and choose those that are closer to feminine sensitivity, such as fashion designing or hairdressing. However, the father's energy remains a universal factor that supports the functioning of each person regardless of his sex or sexual orientation.

Monica ran a company as a franchisee, but the business did not prosper. Interestingly, she had numerous business meetings, the customers were interested in the offer and there were initial arrangements, but eventually they backed out. The constellation showed that the customers wanted to turn to the franchisor and franchisee as a whole. They opened their arms to embrace both companies. Facing only Monica's company, they got discouraged and turned away. It seemed that there should be close communication between the companies, and Monica should not act as an independent business entity.

Monica understood this situation; however, it did not explain everything. When she stood opposite the representative of the franchisor, she could not look up at him. This implied a transference of the attitude from some other relationship. I asked about the relationship with her father. Monica replied, "Now it's okay, we accept each other." It was not the answer indicating that there were no problems in that relationship. I stood as the father, and Monica felt an impulse to crouch, she wanted to accept the hierarchy and the father as a father.

That was what she had lacked to establish a proper relationship with the franchisor and to deal with the customers as a person closely cooperating with that company, which is, after all, the essence of this type of business. Rejecting her place in the parent-child hierarchy resulted in the inability to be in an appropriate relationship with the main company and made the clients confused. It is amazing, but—as one can see—customers are a perfect indicator of disorder.

Often during a constellation, people realize that their relationship with a supervisor or a senior coworker reflects their relationship with the mother or father. In a situation, where we do not have an orderly relationship with our parents, the conflicting aspects of this relationship may manifest themselves at work. A disordered relationship with the parents—in the form of longstanding grievances, rivalry, anger, or negation of relationships—results in a deterioration of our ability to achieve success. Why does this happen? There are two direct causes: lack of strength and self-sabotage. Without feeling our roots, we do not have the strength that flows from our entire family through the parents. We can also sabotage our work ourselves, in order to atone for the inappropriate attitude toward our parents. If, for example, someone graduated from college to prove something to his parents, show that he is better than them, then it may be that he will feel weak and incompetent in his work.

Accepting parents and the ability to feel their presence behind our back (in the metaphorical sense, but partly also in the sensual one) is a great support during our career. Assländer writes that it is easy to see that people who are "conflicted with parents and filled with anger at what the parents did to them will not achieve professional success" (Grün and Assländer 2009, 124).[5]

Charles wanted to "be given back" what he had invested in order to "finally have income from work." He said he was not interested in wealth, but wanted to live normally and have a stable financial situation. He repeatedly asked, quasi-rhetorically, why it kept happening to him, why he still had no money. When he described his situation, it seemed obvious: he found a bad associate, the regulations changed, and he ran into debt. It was as if he wanted the fate to pay for just the effort, regardless of its effects. He was raised by adoptive parents, and when he was coming into his own, he had some ideas and wanted to change jobs, they suggested that he stick to what he had; they were fearful and did not support him. They also left him nothing when they died. It was not until I asked him that he admitted he had a grudge against them. During the constellation, he could face this grudge. In cases such as that of Charles, it is important to realize that one comes from a different family system, so one cannot expect the adoptive parents to satisfy the deep needs that are actually directed to the biological parents. When Charles realized this, he said he felt torn, "I can't leave these, I can't approach those." The solution for him was to internally thank the adoptive parents and gradually approache the biological parents. Then he could fully go into his own life. Feel that he has everything that is necessary to work and achieve success. Charles said that he "had chosen the wrong associates," which could be referred to the adoptive parents. In a sense, they were the "wrong associates" in achieving his sense of strength and professional effectiveness, because for this he needed the connection with his real parents.

Jack worked in the financial sector. When he brought his marker nearer to the financial company marker, he felt that it was turning away. Then he said, "Now I have the impression that they only want to use my knowledge and don't want the rest." I said to him, "Yes, they don't want the rest. But what is the rest? These are a child's desires." Jack: "Yes, I see it now, I didn't say it, but I was attracted by the fact that there would be someone above me there, like a father."

As for his real father, Jack had the impression during the constellation that he was against him. That he even wanted to attack him. But he did not mean the son. I put "something that was related to the father, what he was really looking at." Jack immediately moved it to the middle of the table, between the money, work, and the marker representing himself. He said he felt disgusted with it, then he corrected himself and said he just did not want to have anything to do with it, because it was aggressive. I saw it a bit differently, as something heavy rather than aggressive.

I added a representation of the father's father, and it actually turned out that it was the grandfather who was connected with that "something." I had the impression that it concerned many people, almost like I saw them crammed into the marker. I asked the client if it could be something related to war. He replied that his grandfather had been in the Home Army. He probably had merits and was respected. He did not say much, but he said, "They had to fight, it was the right thing to do."

Jack's job was to leave with respect what belongs to the past, and what subconsciously influenced him and moderated his attitude to his father. It was not without the sense of emptiness, which is—as I already mentioned—frequent in such situations. Then I put the client's marker in the string with the father and grandfather. This gave him greater strength in his relation to work. But Jack felt still "uncertain of his father." The solution would be to say, "It's difficult for me to do what I intend to do without your blessing, without your approval"; "But because I accept you as my father, I will do it." However, Jack was not able to accept his father fully.

At the end of the next constellation, with a group, there was Jack's representative, a representative of masculine strength, a representative of his inner child, and a representative of the father. The representative of Jack's inner child felt that Jack was rejecting him, refusing to accept him. It was only after a long work, when all the mentioned representatives sat close together in a circle, that Jack said, surprised, that something in him was "letting go" and that "he smiled internally" for the first time. Then he could also look at his father for the first time, which was a huge step, considering how intransigent he had been in his aversion to him.

Accepting Life and Accepting Success

It is not true that we all want success and can accept it. It was already Freud who observed that one's reaction to success does not need to be positive. He gave an example of an academic teacher who, after hearing that he could get his dream job, began to depreciate his merits, and finally became depressed. Freud wrote:

> Psychoanalytic work teaches that the forces of conscience which induce illness in consequence of success, instead of, as normally, in consequence of frustration, are closely connected with the Oedipus complex, the relation to father and mother—as perhaps, indeed, is all our sense of guilt in general. (Freud 1957, 331)

According to Manfred Kets de Vries, psychoanalyst and business advisor, one of the explanations for this phenomenon is that:

> [. . .] for some people success becomes equated with a symbolic victory of doing better than the parents of childhood. This is particularly true for those individuals who have never satisfactorily resolved rivalrous feelings toward parents and siblings. (Kets de Vries 2006, 163)

Constellations show that if we have feelings of grievance, jealousy, rivalry, anger, or pain toward the family, achieving success will be difficult. These feelings will use our mental energy and there will not be enough of it for external activities. At the same time, we will not really want success because our deeper desires will, in their entirety, be involved in the management of guilt, anger, and grievance.

In constellations, we can directly test our attitude to success. When someone faces a representative of his success, he may find out that he does not feel ready to come close. It may be that success terrifies him. Why? Because success takes possession, and one has to give oneself up to it. We never fully have our success under control. Success, after all, is never just our success—it always takes place in some environment, in a system of relationships. Every success is a concrete path, which means abandoning other paths, and those who want to feel free will be afraid of it. However, if we avoid success, do we achieve freedom? Of course not. We give up the freedom we can have in favor of the one we can only dream of. Success is also "more"—more activities, contacts, money, work, and responsibility. But perhaps we have created our identity as someone who has little? Maybe if we have little, we feel that we are innocent and we can belong to the family? Maybe someone in the family had little and we identify with him?

Some people want to succeed but do not accept their lives. They want another one. Sometimes they camouflage it by saying that they want to change their lives. But can one change anything rejecting it at the same time?

Lisa said she took too much on herself and eventually had enough of everything. I did not need a lot of information, as it was clear that it was difficult for her to take. This suggested the interrupted movement of love, and indeed, in the constellation, Lisa's representative was greatly distanced from the mother. I asked if there were any events in her life that involved separation from the mother. It turned out that Lisa, as a two-year-old child, had been hospitalized three times for operations for a deformed lip and that the operations had failed. Lisa confessed, "I hate the whole world." As she spoke, I felt compassion for her inner child. Something became clear to me, so I said, "You've only thought about your lip all your life and showed it to everyone." Lisa: "Oh yes, and my family, sisters, talked about it too." It was anger and rebellion of a child. Lisa never accepted her life; she rejected it all the more because she felt separated from her mother. Using her defect, she blamed both her mother and the world.

Was she able to attain any success in that way? She did not want it; she even hated it. However, she wanted to work on it and change it. She had to accept her mother, her life, her body, and the world around her. What could she start with? With gratitude for her life.

Money and Work

Money is related to giving and taking. That is why it is not something static and permanent; it is movement. However, money has a long history, which makes it real too. One cannot escape money, although many would like to. Money seems to be something dirty and bad to them, regardless of the fact that they want it at a conscious level. Why is money badly associated?

Perhaps contact with money brings hidden secrets, deceptions, injustices, and harms from the past out of the subconsciousness?

There are many unconscious dynamics connected with money. For example, falling into debt as a result of taking loans may result from the interrupted bond and inability to take from the mother. In such cases, credits mean love and care. Sometimes families embroil themselves in debts over generations, and these debts are just a reflection of the lack of order on the emotional plane. They result from the transmission and escalation of effects of some bond lost in the past. Money is to bring it back, but it cannot do it. Such money "in place of something" will never suffice and will never bring satisfaction.

A common problem related by the clients is financial loss, regular bankruptcy, or inability to collect debts; they are unable to maintain liquidity or are "in the red." In such cases, losses caused by an entanglement may be involved. By losing money, we try to compensate someone whose fate is perceived by us as harm. As if we donated our money to him. The solution here is to get to know this mechanism, see the person and take him into the heart, and leave his fate with respect.

We may also have difficulties in taking. An example is the case of Amelia, who, despite being able to establish various businesses and earn, still had no money, always lost it. The short constellation, in which I stood as a representative of her mother, showed that it was difficult for her to take. She could give but could not take.

With the help of money, we may want to repair a damage that was done in previous generations. Yvonne, who was enmeshed in her husband's great debts and who always "took everything on her shoulders," in fact wanted to do something for her great-grandfather. The great-grandfather's representative uttered the following words, "We're finished," "This land won't yield anymore," "Everything's gone." There seemed to be some great loss that plunged the family. The great-grandfather was a farmer, it was during the war. The great-granddaughter, working for her husband and taking on the debts incurred by him, in some way connected with her great-grandfather's hard lot.

When we see new opportunities related to finance, profession, or self-fulfillment, we sometimes lose sight of our roots. We do not remember the past, and we want to happily enter the future. To our surprise, this does not work. There are fears, a blockage within us, or an external obstacle. Why does this happen? It is in this form that a bond with someone from our past is manifested. Very often, to succeed, we must recognize that we are not going to do it alone. The idea "me and my goal" is not enough. We need to include someone else in this arrangement. This may be not only the former business partner or founder of the company but also the dead siblings or aborted child, sometimes the ex-partner. It is only when we give them a place in our heart that we begin to deserve success. To deserve in the eyes of our unconscious conscience. When this is done, in a sense, success is ours if we just work hard enough for it.

When we close ourselves internally and want to gain by excluding people from our lives and trying not to remember our history, we become closed and unable to succeed. And if we do succeed, for example, on the financial level, we often have to pay with our health or a worsening of our relationships.

Nancy wanted to establish a company with two business partners. Actually three, because—as she said—a wife of one of them was also initially involved in the business, but later gave birth to a child and withdrew. She was not supposed to actively influence the enterprise; she was just to be formally present in it. Apart from this married couple, an older man, whom Nancy had known for years, was to join the company. Very pragmatic, interested only in the business side of the venture. The client said, however, that something kept her from building the company, despite she was keen on this idea.

I asked Nancy to set up the constellation using plastic markers. The elements that appeared in the constellation were the client, the company, the older man, the young man, and his wife. After a while, I added the profit (money) marker. When I did that, Nancy wanted to remove her marker from the table and moved it to the very edge. The wife's reaction was interesting, as she was attracted to the profit. Nancy made a comment: "She feels the joy of a little girl." The older man was also interested in the profit, but in a more calm and controlled way. The young man was kind of shy, insecure; he seemed to wait for his wife to decide.

Seeing the wife's attitude, I set up her mother behind her. The daughter had an unclear attitude toward the mother. Then the client told me a story related to that woman's family. Her father, after his mother's death, was raised by his stepmother, she also took care of his siblings. She was childless. The children did not accept her. Her husband (father's father) left her land and house in his will. However, as an old woman, she was removed ("taken out") from there, which happened after the woman and man who were to enter the company had become married. The idea to establish the company was born on that land and certain solutions related to its operations were tested there.

I did not analyze and try to understand all the connections and dependencies that existed in this case. However, the client received some important information. She saw that the young woman was determined by her own history, she noticed the dependence of the young man on his wife, as well as her ambiguous attitude to the money that was to come from the business. Such knowledge, without further directing the client and without giving advice, causes change itself.

We look at the property and inheritance we receive, and the real property we own as pure profit. However, these things are systemically connected, they are an element or visible trace of the fate of people along with the disorder in which they were involved, and the tragedies that hit them. Do we also accept our family heritage when taking the parent's inheritance? Or do we only take the money and exclude the testator from our hearts? Do we take the inherited house as a visible sign of our belonging to the family and do we want to pass it on to our children along with the memory of their grandparents, the people from whom we got it? Or do we take the credit? When we inherit, do we treat ourselves in the same way as our siblings?

Much depends on the answers to the above questions. Many would do better if they gave up their struggle for inheritance and agreed on what comes to them itself. Money obtained without respect for the donor destroys the holder from the inside. How many people suffered a life failure after they had taken money they could not thank for? They quickly lost it, not feeling entitled to have it. The money taken out of disorder only worsens it. Unconsciously, we desire to get rid of it or lose it, feeling that we do not deserve it.

Money comes from our work, our profession. A profession is a social identity and place in society. Hellinger says that a place:

> [. . .] makes sense when it is one of many. No one has a place just for themselves. We occupy our place with many others who are next to us. We also dispute each other's places and yet we are dependent on the fact that the others occupy their place. How else could we make an exchange with them, take from them and give to them. (Hellinger 2011, 18)[6]

We constantly occupy and vacate our places; we do it by changing professions, jobs, or by leaving this world. We alternately compete and cooperate with others. As Hellinger says, in the end, it "is about getting a better place, even the best place for our survival," "it is a matter of life and death" (Hellinger 2011, 18)[7]. This is probably why work is so strongly connected with the deep dynamics of life and family, in which our survival is also at stake.

Work is a big part of man's life. It defines his identity, it connects with the history of the family, country, and humanity. Many unconscious factors influence his choice. It seems that some of us, when choosing a profession, are particularly strongly motivated by something that lies beyond their consciousness. Among such people there are real enthusiasts, devoted to very useful activities: helping the disabled, saving animals, medical, or *pro publico bono* activities. Many of them fulfill themselves in these activities for the benefit of other people.

Often, by choosing some profession associated with treatment, we want to help someone in the family, for instance, the mother. People who become physicians or nurses often patronize their parents. They want to be independent of any need for care and occupy the highest place in the family hierarchy. The same applies to psychotherapists who often want to save someone from the distant past. On the other hand, those who choose law or service in the police may be motivated by a desire to repair some old family injustice, by a need to restore order.

It happens that the chosen occupation, although desired, does not bring satisfaction. The person feels that the anxiety that drives him does not go away. Then he cannot enjoy the effects of his useful work. Suzanne founded and ran a foundation that helped the disabled. The activity proved to be useful and was esteemed. However, she did not get rid of the sense of meaninglessness—after all, so many people suffer, she could not help everyone, how could she live with that? In an individual constellation, as a representative of her father, I felt mental pain. As her grandfather—I felt something similar, but there was also a strange move: I stretched one hand to the side and slightly up, and the other one down. There I put a sheet of paper marked as "something that matters here." It looked as if I tried to grab something with my hand held up and catch someone with the other. A fleeting vision of a train carriage came to my mind. The client picked up on the thought, saying that in her grandfather's life there was some work associated with railway. The constellation showed that there had been a tragic event in which the grandfather had participated and probably blamed himself for not being able to help someone. His son and then his grand-daughter, Suzanne, were connected with that story and the victim. That is why she felt that her life and work did not make sense, because she "could not help everyone."

NOTES

1. Quotation translated from Polish.
2. Quotation translated from Polish.
3. Quotation translated from German.
4. Quotation translated from German.
5. Quotation translated from Polish.
6. Quotation translated from German.
7. Quotation translated from German.

Chapter 11

Development of Disorders and Problems—Metaprocesses

DIFFICULTIES IN ACCEPTING LIFE

In previous chapters, the reader could familiarize himself with the theory and elements of the constellation therapist's work. I showed how system dynamics create or cocreate psychophysical, interpersonal, or professional problems. It turns out that in all these areas, similar factors and patterns play a role. We can understand them as the dynamics of belonging and exclusion, hidden bonds, loyalty, unconscious activity of conscience that aims at balancing through atonement, and unconscious violation of the system hierarchy.

I present the disturbing processes under several main categories: difficulties in accepting life, parents, and the strength of the family, transgenerational burdens, and perinatal difficulties. These categories are not separable and overlap in many places. In this chapter, I also present my own concept of the so-called systemic-psychodynamic transduction, which I consider to be a very important—although so far completely unknown—process that shapes character as well as persistent and difficult to change mental disorders.

Let us start from the beginning—the question of accepting one's own life. Sessions of systemic constellations show very clearly that there are varying "degrees of acceptance of one's life." Accepting life is not obvious. We settle for our lives, want these lives, and are grateful for them to different degrees. Saying "Yes" to one's life is essential to being healthy and feeling good. The problem is that we may not know whether we say "Yes" or rather "No" to our life internally. For this process is partly hidden from our consciousness. In constellations, it comes to light, thanks to which we can change our attitude.

Based on my own experience, Hellinger's work, Mark Wolynn's findings (Wolynn 2016, 63), and the Austermanns' observations (Austermann and

Austermann 2019), I can list the following motives that disrupt the flow of life:

- An interruption of the early bond with the mother;
- Rejecting a parent;
- Symbiosis with a parent;
- A feeling of guilt and strong attempt to make up to the mother;
- Identification with someone from the family system (entanglement);
- The existence of a dead twin;
- Deep dissatisfaction with one's fate.

As one can see, basically, all the problems we encounter during constellations are related to difficulty in "accepting life" or difficulty in "living one's own life." The point is, however, that perinatal problems and an early interruption of the bond with the mother can result in rejection of life on the most fundamental level.

Symbiosis or merging with a parent makes it impossible to direct oneself toward one's own life. Behind symbiosis, there is always rejection of the parent. In order to accept him with gratitude one must first stand—internally—face to face with him, and this in a symbiotic state is impossible. As there is no conscious acceptance, the unconscious entanglement in the parent figure, in his feelings and problems deepens. That is why symbiosis is a kind of vicious circle. The symbiotic problem is likely to affect mothers and daughters to the greatest extent.

A sense of guilt can be an obstacle to taking one's life. Feeling guilty is common in those who survived the Holocaust or great catastrophes. It is difficult for those people to live. Also, children may feel guilty about their mother and not fully take the life they have been given.

Zoe felt guilty about her mother's illness that had developed after the delivery (infection and development of diabetes). That is why it was hard for her to take the life that her mother had given her and be happy. She wanted a balance to be brought about. However, in the constellation, the mother's representative considered this attitude to be inappropriate. A child must say to his mother, "I take the life you gave me. At the price you and I had to pay. I will make good use of my life." The mother did not want a compensation through atonement from the child, she felt that the price she paid was her concern. However, it was difficult for the daughter to leave it with her mother. Thus, she did not take the place that was appropriate for the child. She tried to break out of the one-way flow and give back "against the current," rather than say, "I am just a child. I can only take from you."

Finally, Zoe said she took her life and thanked her mother for it, but she added, "I won't let you down." Thereby she returned to the starting point—she showed that she would not give up the balancing (there is this sentence of strength: "I will make something of my life in memory of you," but something else was said in this case). It was the activity of the primary conscience that orders us to give back when we received, to lose when we caused someone to lose. When she finally confronted the fact that this was not the way, she said with tears, "I'm afraid of loneliness." Only after a long work did she feel that she could thank her mother, take her into the heart, and turn to her own life.

Giving the mother her responsibility back and taking one's own life is a step toward independence. It always entails risk of loneliness. The attempts to pay the mother back entangled the client in the exchange game, which protected her from that feeling.

We are separated from life by entanglements in other system members, often unknown to us. When we are unconsciously connected with someone, whose fate was harsh, who died early, or was abandoned, we do not accept our own life. We do not live it. It stands next to us. By discovering the entanglement and taking that person into the heart, we return to our lives, which has concrete psychophysical effects in the form of improved health and mood.

The cases presented by the Austermanns show that having unknown twin siblings may prevent one from taking one's life completely and with gratitude. Since one of the twins died, the one who survived does not feel fully entitled to enjoy his own life.

Another factor separating from life is lack of acceptance of fate. This kind of lack of acceptance does not only concern fate, it always involves disrupted relations with members of the system.

Thirty-year-old Mary, the oldest of three siblings, said that she was attached to her mother too much, that she wanted to get some independence. She did not start a family, as she felt that she had to be with the mother all the time, because she expected her support. She anticipated the mother's needs in advance fearing her criticism and dissatisfaction. I presumed that was due to the interrupted movement of love, which was confirmed by the constellation. Mary was born with a serious leg defect, the birth was difficult, and the baby was shown to the mother with a considerable delay. The constellation also revealed that the mother was unconsciously bound to someone, which escalated her partial unavailability for the child.

However, something else was particularly interesting here. Mary's representative, and then herself, rebelled and wanted the mother to love her more than the rest of the siblings. It was quite surprising—it was not that she got less, she clearly demanded more. Why? It was in this way that her disability was to be compensated by the mother. It seemed as if to her the mother was her fate, so she was responsible for the handicap. Probably on the subconscious level, every child sees his mother as the one who answers for everything and can do anything. In this case, certain sentences of strength led her to take from the mother what the mother really gave and to give up the unreasonable desires. Mary's task was to abandon the fantasy of the mother-fate, the mother-god who was expected to pay for the harm, and to open herself to take from the mother who gave as much as she could. It was the way to accept her fate and life.

CUTTING OFF FROM PARENTS AND THE STRENGTH OF ANCESTORS

Cutting Off from Parents—External Factors

Someone who has not accepted his mother or father, regardless of what they were like, lives with a lowered life energy level, and this energy level is further lowered as a result of internal tensions associated with separation from the parents. People with this problem often experience depressive states and difficulties in their own life, health problems, not to mention various problems in relationships.

It seems that rejecting a parent always has some external cause, but it continues due to the inner attitude. A good internal relationship with the parents is also hindered by situations involving serious parental negligence, abandonment of the child, the parent's alcoholism, physical or mental illness, serious crimes committed by the parent (e.g., murder), and his early death. These events often lead to an early form of isolation from the parent, which is the interrupted primal movement toward the parent. Sending the child away to his grandparents for upbringing in the first years of life also results in problems with accepting the mother or father. Importantly, these primal forms of internal distance from the parents often remain unconscious.

The difficulties in accepting the parents—manifested in resentment, disrespect, and rejecting them—at a later age take place when one parent excludes, disrespects, or judges the other. It is difficult for the child to accept not only the disrespected parent but also the one who excludes. The child painfully, though often unconsciously, feels the harm that is done to the other parent. In addition, he feels that the parent's anger is also directed against him, even if the parent swears it is not. The son cannot share the mother's negative opinion about the father. How would he do that without aggression directed at himself? After all, he also comes from him and has a part in him that is related to the father. Like the father, he is a man. And yet many sons do this. They remain weak and torn. They hate their mothers internally, and they do not know anything about this hatred. It is transferred onto their partners or their body and health.

So how could the child attacked at such a deep level accept his mother? The mother's anger rarely results solely from what happened between her and the father. It is generally rooted in the system of origin. Like everything that is intense and does not fade with time. The son can look at his mother's attitude from this perspective: it is not really about my father.

The difficulties for the child also arise when the parents find it hard to feel that they are a couple. This may be the case when the child is the result of an accidental encounter; when the father and mother did not love each other and never lived together. In a constellation, their representatives can look at each other, so that it becomes clear for the child that "they were together enough to become parents." In this way, the parental couple, that has in fact existed since conception, is constituted in the consciousness of the child. Ultimately, the couple's child needs to recognize that he has parents, "just like everyone else." He must leave the idea that he "has no" father or mother. The same applies to the child conceived as a result of rape.

Also the child who is committed to fixing his parents' marriage or "arranging" their divorce loses his parents as parents. The result is a difficulty in taking care of his own life. By violating the system hierarchy between the "earlier" and the "later," the child gains an apparent sense of agency toward his parents and loses real effectiveness in his own life. Externally, these are often very "adult" people, but with a child underneath.

The parent makes it impossible for the child to be close to him also when he projects something onto the child that has nothing to do with the latter—he sees his ex-partner or parent in the child, or he locates in him the emotions and matters of the family's past, from which he himself turns away. The child, driven by love, tries to take guilt away from the parent, replace his parents, or save his life if the parent seeks death internally. However, such love-driven actions are also an obstacle to accepting the parent. For the child is absorbed in his affairs, but isolated from him. The real acceptance of the parent can only take place if the child opens up to the parent as a parent and leaves his affairs with him.

The child distances himself also from the parent who does not accept his parents, or his grandparents. Such a child automatically isolates himself. In the constellation, we see that when we help the father or mother—thanks to the representatives—to accept their own parents, their child also opens up to them.

Cutting Off from Parents—Internal Factors

The factors I referred to as "external" trigger or strengthen internal mechanisms that stand in the way of approaching one's parents. It is amazing, but practice shows how easily a child can turn away from his parent. The child does not see and take into account the determinants of his emotions and behavior, and additionally looks at him from an egocentric perspective. He believes that everything the parent does or says in his presence relates to him. It is also characteristic that we remember negative events, usually without noticing the daily labor of our parents. Who of us remembers that our mother lacked sleep and was tired when we cried during the day and woke up at night as infants? Who knows and thinks about the father's difficulties related to the financial side of our coming into the world? These actions undertaken by our parents, directed at our survival, remain forever in the shadows.

Accepting the parent is therefore hindered by judging him. The child only seemingly judges the parent fairly. When judging their parents, the children are always mistaken because they never know the wider context. How much are we really told about the past of the family and parents? Moreover, the full context is not known by the parents themselves, as they too are unaware of the past events that have affected them.

There are extreme situations, but usually a significant number of grievances against the parents turn out to be excessive. Even if the parents are bad for their children, the question is why they are bad. However, the child does not ask that. The child's thinking is that the parent does what he does because he wants to. The parent is the master of his own life and the master of the child's life. How many people do not see that—judging their parents—they think like children?

Another internal mechanism that makes it difficult to be closer to the parent is the sense of justice. Some people find it hard to take a step toward reconciliation and love, as this would prevent them from seeking redress. They expect their parents to pay, apologize, or "plead guilty." Of course, it can be that the parents deny certain facts or their inappropriate behavior. Sometimes we have to agree to this (although constellations enable us to discover the most important facts, such as having unknown siblings). It is necessary to leave the difficulty in "standing in the truth" with the parents. Otherwise, we will not even notice when "justice" becomes more important to us than our life and success.

Sometimes the problems with accepting the parent result from persistent infantile jealousy and fantasies. Complaining about the parent "favoring" one's sibling is one of the most popular in this category. The parents are described as cold, and all their merits seem to mean nothing compared to this. As for those "favored" and "ignored," I noticed one common pattern. The favored one almost always fares worse than the allegedly ignored one. There is nothing surprising about this. The favored ones were most often spoiled and not controlled. On the other hand, they were often burdened with unfulfilled desires of their parents. From the ignored, something was required and the results of their actions were checked. The first were not taught and basically left alone to do whatever they wanted, the latter were taught something. So what worked to the detriment in the lives of the first is seen as desired by the second—without considering the facts at all.

Violating the hierarchy and looking down on the parents is also a source of being cut off from the strength that flows from them. It can be camouflaged. Frequently, behind positive actions, such as helping parents with their affairs, there is an attitude of towering over them. Such children exalt themselves, although outwardly it only looks like care for the infirm parents. In particular, the child who had to take care of himself too quickly, and sometimes also help the parents, will tend to look down on them. Such children do not take their parents seriously. Therefore, they will lose them even more.

It happens that an older sister "replaces" the mother and looks after her siblings. She feels that it is her job since the mother is incapable. This attitude in adulthood is not good for anyone. In fact, it closes the access to the real mother for both this sister and her siblings. Although the situation of premature responsibility was not comfortable and its consequences are not good at all, in adulthood, it is difficult to give up the inner attitude of superiority. It is a feeling of being someone better, which results from the idea that one has always been independent and grown up.

Cutting Off from the Family

Internal separation from parents blocks the flow of strength from the family. The strength that flows to us from our ancestors is not a myth and everyone can experience it during constellations. The problem is that it is often blocked. This blockage results, on the one hand, from systemic disorder in the family and, on the other hand, from the attitude of the given person.

Pauline lacked energy, joy of life, a sense of who she was and what she wanted, and any satisfaction with her sex life. When she stood in front of the pyramid of her family—sheets of paper marked accordingly represented her mother, father, grandparents, and great-grandparents—it was obvious that she needed to feel connected with them and open up to taking strength from her ancestors so that something in her life could change.

She felt, however, that she wanted to cut off from them all, that she wanted to "decide about her life" by herself. They had always had some expectations from her, to which she had subordinated herself. To help the client and better understand her state, I started representing her myself. Only then did I see how deep her separation from the family was. When I looked at the pieces of paper representing the family, I felt nothing positive. Instead, I had the impression that they were all looking at me and expecting something, and even more, as if they had collected some of their problems together to burden me with them. As Pauline, I absolutely did not feel like the fruit of the family and someone who has the full right to go to their own life, with the support of their ancestors behind. What I felt was fear and weakness and I sat on the floor. I asked Pauline to sit next to me. I felt that I wanted to fuse with her, to be embraced by her. I asked what she felt, if she felt distanced from the person I represented. Pauline confirmed. I represented a part of her, from which she had cut herself off.

In the further part of the constellation, Pauline said that when she was a child her parents told her she did not match their family, they complained that it was as if she had been from another family. Pauline did not know what they meant. Just like when her friends told her that even though they knew her for so long, they did not really know what she was like. I saw an outline of a certain mechanism here. A long time ago, as a small child, in order to protect herself, to survive mentally, she detached herself from part of her personality. She was not able to go into her own life "entirely," because she had to leave behind the "part" that felt burdened by her ancestors. So she was left with no energy and no clear sense of identity. At the same time, she wanted to break away from the family even more.

One could say that there is such a thing as "fear of the family," which makes some people feel they need to run away from it instead of taking strength from it. They are not only cut off from their father or mother, but from both parents and the entire family. These people live as if they wanted to start all over again—without memories, without bonds, without memorabilia, and photographs. It is a difficult fate, as entanglements and hidden loyalties cannot be removed by "cutting oneself off." Nor can one have full strength without the ancestors behind one's back. Then one loses a part of the parental, social, and professional competence. One loses a part of the ability to coexist with the opposite sex. One loses a part, or even a lot, of vitality and health.

TRANSGENERATIONAL BURDENS

Transgenerational Trauma

Much has been written about traumas, but do we know everything about their nature? It is not at all obvious what traumatizes and how it happens. If someone barely escaped from a burning building in which his loved ones died, it will be a great trauma for him. There are also less obvious traumas. A young girl can experience a trauma when seeing her boyfriend's arousal. Why? The level of trauma depends not only on external circumstances but also on the individual's inner world. What will be a lifelong shock to one, someone else will quickly forget. Constellations shed light on this phenomenon too, showing the deeper mechanisms of traumatic influences.

When Greta's husband screamed at her, she froze as if paralyzed, afraid to speak. She associated this with a situation when she was three to five years old at most. To get her parents' attention, she cut off a lock of her hair. Her father went crazy and smashed the table on the floor, ad the mother told her to sit quietly. Greta was terrified. I said that since this situation continued to affect her, she apparently stuck to it herself.

When I stood as Greta's father, I felt the energy of the perpetrator—my fists clenched, I wanted to shake them and hit. Greta mentioned then that her father's father "fought in two wars." I stood as the grandfather. I felt a kind of nausea (Greta said she also suffered from it), my eyelids clenched, and I felt alarmed. It was as if the grandfather had witnessed or caused something disgusting, something he did not want to look at. I placed two objects on the floor representing the persons with whom the grandfather was connected. When that bond was shown, Greta felt relieved. Then I stood as the father again. Only now was it easier for her to look at him. But there was still something wrong. I added an item representing the father's mother. It was very difficult for the father to accept his parents because he wanted to be someone special to his mother. When I finally managed, as the father's representative, to say to his mother without inner resistance or hesitation, "I'm just a child," Greta could also stand comfortably in front of her father and say to him, "I'm just a child." Some time after the constellation she said that she felt very well and was more "like a woman" for her husband. I said that now she knew "with whom she was a child and with whom she was a woman."

This constellation tells us something about the nature of trauma. In this case, the real trauma was not that the father shouted and smashed the table, but his inner attitude, which he had brought into the relationship with his daughter. He carried in himself the energy of the perpetrator taken over from the previous generation and a tangle of roles—of the mother's son and partner. What did it cause? It caused his daughter to see incomprehensible aggression and anger as well as incestuous eroticism in him. It was this mixture that was traumatic rather than the father's behavior. As an adult, Greta chose a husband who paralyzed her by screaming and, as I know from another constellation, had an overly intimate relationship with the daughter.

Something becomes traumatic if it has not been mentally controlled and incorporated into the circulation of conscious thoughts, as it turned out to be too strong, too difficult for that. This is a classic concept of trauma, originated by Josef Breuer and Sigmund Freud. Constellations add one basic detail here. The contents and affects, that are not included in conscious thinking, not only accumulate in the unconscious but remain as if outside the mind. They become an unbearable emotional element that "lives between" the family members. This trauma status that goes beyond the individual is the cause of its transmission to the next generations.

Facilitating constellations, I came across several major types of events that have dramatic effects on the next generations. These are death of a child, death of a woman in childbirth, murders, abortions (especially multiple and without afterthought), mass war deaths, but also early orphanhood, or concealment of paternity, for example, when the child was the result of infidelity or rape. In the latter case, several generations suffer from a social morality that unduly stigmatizes such situations. The ancestor who was a rapist becomes excluded and forgotten, but the souls of his children and grandchildren demand his acceptance. This is quite obvious, because they are influenced by the order requiring to thank him for life. They cannot do so, however, because the ancestor's place on their inner family tree is empty. This causes that they do not have full life force and do not allow themselves to be happy.

When the parent, the father or mother dies, it is a great trauma for the child, because of which—and because of his mental immaturity—he is unable to go through mourning. He shuts away from pain, grief, fear, and anger. This is a classic example of repression—as an adult, he may feel that nothing serious has happened. This stems from the fact that he has not experienced mourning, that is, that he has not fully felt and mentally and emotionally worked through the loss. However, the energy of loss, as we could call the whole complex of repressed and suppressed feelings, continues in him and influences his life. It also affects the next generations.

In the case of one of my clients, Kenneth, the consequences of losing the father continued for four generations. Kenneth's father lost his father when he was nine years old. All his life he felt resentment due to the lack of the father, Kenneth sometimes saw him cry. What did this result in for Kenneth? The grandfather did not exist for him. He had no place in his heart, for he was someone who was "missing," who was lost. It was only in the constellation that Kenneth felt, to his surprise, a bond with his grandfather, he saw him as a "good person, a being." The constellation also showed that the grandfather identically experienced the relationship with his father—as if he had lost him completely. The client felt that someone else was also important here. So we added his great-grandfather. The great-grandfather was too cut off from his father. When in the constellation, all these men found their way to their fathers, and the sequence of generations was renewed, Kenneth felt great relief and strength.

Sexual abuse manifests itself in constellations as a broad interpersonal and multigenerational system. The mother of Lucy, who was molested in her childhood, seemed to be indifferent to the child's trauma, and even more—her representative said, "Something about this turns me on, these sadomasochistic issues have always been present in our family." Also, a whip and perverse sexual activities came to her mind. When I set up another representative, he felt he was a soldier. The client said that the Russians had entered the village where her grandmother had lived and had raped women. The next representative had sexual impulses directed at the representative of her grandmother, who had been a child during the war. The words "Now us, the lords" came to his mind. The client said that the grandmother and her parents had lived in a manor house and the Russians "had felt at home there." To conclude, Lucy's mother was deeply traumatized, but it was not a personal trauma, but a trauma taken over from her mother. So she adopted a strong, even a bit violent attitude, as the client described her, and was unable to adequately react to her child's harm. Perhaps she expected her daughter not to cause problems, to be strong like her, and imagined that in this way both of them would resist the traumas of the past.

Cecilia said she wanted to work on her failed relationships with men. It was hard for her, however, to articulate what she actually meant—she had a lump in her throat, she was trembling. She confessed that at the age of about 12 she had been sexually abused by her brother, one year older than herself. The other brother was reportedly fascinated by this and supported the younger brother. During the constellation, Cecilia's representative was afraid of the molesting brother's representative. I asked myself the seemingly inappropriate question: "Why this fear?" Then the representatives began to show that there was fascination and love between the brother and sister; that there was an aspect of fun in what they were doing; that they were a kind of married couple. The latter was spontaneously confirmed by Cecilia. I also brought in the mother, the father, the other brother, and then "sexuality, eroticism, what was between the parents" ("eroticism"). The mother was cold and had no erotic connection with the father. I asked Cecilia if her mother was critical of sex. Cecilia confirmed, sex was a taboo subject in their home. So what was Cecilia afraid of? She was afraid of being rejected by her mother—she was afraid she would do something that would separate her from the mother.

I positioned the mother's mother and father. The mother's father felt he wanted to "show something there" to his daughter, something that came from the past and was associated with sexuality. On the other hand, the mother's mother wanted to protect her daughter from this and separate her from the father. Then I set up a representative for "that something from the past." The representative had very strong feelings, fell to the floor with his legs open, started to howl and cry. It became clear to everyone that this was a raped woman. Soon both the representative of the raped woman and the representative of Cecilia became convinced that there was a child in the raped woman's womb. I added a representative of the rapist. After some time, the raped woman, child, and rapist formed a separate circle. The others looked at them and then bowed before them and their fate as the thing that affected the whole family.

I asked the raped woman to say to "eroticism," "I accept you." This was not the end, however. Cecilia, who was already in the constellation in person, said it was better, but she did not feel it was a complete solution. I asked her to stand in front of "eroticism." She could not look the representative in the eye, she felt there was "something dirty" there that she could not take. "Eroticism" felt it was good and would give Cecilia strength and energy. It was the moment of work with the client's inner attitude. The point was to enable the client to free herself from the negative attitude to sexuality. Just because a woman was raped does not mean she is able to reject sexuality. That is why I asked Cecilia to say to "eroticism:" "You are bigger." These words helped her regain the right measure. After all, no one is able to take offense at sexuality, to judge it, to put themselves above or beyond it. In the end, Cecilia felt the connection, hugged the representative of eroticism, feeling that she agreed to sexuality and took its energy.

Considering the issue of transmission of trauma between generations from the perspective of general processes, we can observe the phenomenon of intergenerational transformation and even acceleration of trauma. Trauma does not disappear, nor does it gradually diminish, but over two or three generations its effects may even intensify. Original traumatic events may have a stronger psychological impact on future generations than on their participants. This is due to the fact that what was a temporary event in the life of an adult becomes an element accompanying his child's development from the very beginning. While the parent was affected by the external event, his child is affected by the parent's internal state. And what takes place in the relationship has a stronger psychological impact than purely physical factors.

War as Trauma

Although decades have passed, many causes of the problems of people born in Central or Eastern Europe and in Germany lie in war events. The trauma of genocide and war affects the third and fourth generation—people who are completely unaware of these connections. For example, a man experienced something heavy, related to the Holocaust, but remains calm and withdrawn, he does not talk about it. His daughter unconsciously sees his fragile inner part and takes on herself some of the trauma. Later, she has a daughter, she cannot give herself fully to the daughter and provide her with a sense of security, because she looks at her father's trauma, carrying part of it within herself. Then the daughter has her own child—he is the great-grandson. His upbringing will be marked by the unsatisfactory relationship between his mother and her mother. Will this child ever think that his difficulties are rooted in the events of World War II? He will rather see their cause in his mother's attitude.

It is all a linear transmission, from one person to another. Constellations indicate that there is also a direct connection with the ancestors and the traumas that affected them. The war still has its consequences, the events related to it influence the psyche of subsequent generations. The descendants of those who fought, died and killed, or witnessed the war, take on themselves their pain and emotional withdrawal and also try to unite the perpetrators and their victims.

In the constellation of a client, whose parents were from the vicinity of Minsk in Belarus and Lviv (formerly, Poland, now Ukraine) and her husband's parents were from Germany, there were several dead and at least two killers. It seemed that there were killings in both the father's and mother's lines. There was also a dead woman there, as felt by her representative, probably with a child in her womb. Another representative felt she was holding a knife, threatening a person lying on the floor, as if in an act of revenge. This constellation made me think of the mass murders such as the Volhynian slaughter.[1] The client's son's serious psychological problems, with which the client came, were connected with these traumas. They affected him as if directly (*via* the family field), not through upbringing.

Traumatic events from the past can cause people in the next generations to try not to look back to cut themselves off from the horrifying events. However, because of this, their relationships with their parents and grandparents suffer, they cannot take the strength from them, and negative patterns of family relationships are transmitted to the next generations. In such cases, it is necessary to look at the past, to bow to what determined the fate of the family so strongly, and then to leave the past where it belongs, accept the ancestors, and leave their pain and traumas.

A young man who stuttered since childhood came to one of the workshops. Stuttering is like a combination of speaking and being silent. So at the beginning, the therapist set up "what speaks in him" and "what is silent." The representative of "speaking" made a gesture as if he was shooting the representative of "muteness." The client said then that his great-grandfather had closely collaborated with Józef Piłsudski and fought the Bolsheviks.[2] The great-grandfather, Józef Piłsudski and Russian soldiers were also brought in the constellation. The Russians were strong at first, and then weakened. The great-grandfather aimed at reconciliation, which was completed by his great-grandson, the client. The reconciliation took place when the representatives of "speaking" and "muteness"—or in fact a Pole and a Russian—embraced together with the client. The great-grandfather joined them. There was a moment when the client—following his movement—knelt before Piłsudski's representative. I think that his problem, stuttering, was connected with the need for reconciliation, and also with a sense of loyalty to one side, Poles. It was only when he expressed respect for Piłsudski and saw his great-grandfather's conciliatory movement that he was able to integrate in his soul what was "Polish" with what was "Russian." And thereby resolve his "speaking—not speaking" conflict.

Clara's son suffered from schizophrenia. Her grandfather, a Jewish woman, and war events proved to be important in her constellation. Clara only remembered that her grandfather had gone out to "drive the Jewish woman who had been hiding in a dugout," probably belonging to him. "After two days he came back, changed, from the Gestapo." When I stood as a representative of the person that Clara later identified as her grandfather, I stood upright, raised my chin. I felt the energy of the perpetrator, as I rhythmically clenched my fists. As the grandfather, I turned to the sheet of paper representing Clara's sick son. The grandfather's condition was peculiar. It was a kind of detachment from reality, tension, as if he was clinging to something in himself and isolating himself. Then Clara said that at that time, death threatened the whole family. So the grandfather, doing bad things, in a way did the right thing, he did what he was forced to do. In the constellation, he was unable to reflect on anything, he was internally blocked and restless. As if he was plagued by guilt that he, however, did not allow himself to feel. There was a kind of madness in him. When he lay down next to the objects representing the dead, including the Jewish woman, he reached out his hand in her direction. There was something erotic about it, as if he was caressing her.

After this session, Clara felt freed, she said she was cheerful for the first time in a long time. Before that, when she had gone to bed, she had had thoughts: "Somebody! Get me out of here, save me!" She did not know what she meant then, now she associated the thoughts with the past events. The moral confusion and pain that the grandfather never expressed seems to have been transmitted to the next generations, manifesting themselves in Clara's problems and her son's illness.

Mira had many abortions, one of her babies was premature and died, she also considered aborting her older daughter. This daughter was almost 40 years old when Mira had her constellation; she was a jobless drug addict, full of anger and reproach. She had two abortions herself. The younger daughter had one abortion. Mira's parents and her husband's parents survived the Auschwitz Camp, the war, the escape from the house where they were to be burned. The constellation was dramatic and showed the connection between those who died in the war and the aborted children. The great chaos that reigned in the life of Mira and her family was rooted in the war.

In such situations, bringing in a representative of war helps. Realizing that you were under the influence of forces more powerful than personal choices frees you from guilt, from futile attempts to compensate, and helps you to look differently at the people around you, for example, your parents. The child notices that they were not free, that they were governed by a powerful force that was hidden in the background. War is something that transcends the individual, family, group, and even entire nations. No one "leads" the war once it begins.

I noticed a phenomenon that I could refer to as war trauma of mothers. What happens during a war is unacceptable to a mother—a woman who wants to protect her children at all costs. I have observed that it is particularly difficult for mothers to recognize that there is something they have no influence on, something that even their maternal power must bow to: war in its superhuman dimension. However, war turns out to be beyond simple assimilation, which has transgenerational consequences. No one recognizes the tragic magnitude of war and in the next generations, the daughters see the mothers as guilty, cold, or rejecting. The solution is to accept war as something that transcends the individual. Accepting one's own smallness in its face. When the representatives of the past and present generations can do this, there is relief. Relief in the relationships between the mothers and children. Even those who knew war only from movies.

Transgenerational Guilt

It seems that guilt can be transmitted between generations, especially the one that is repressed and denied. What could be that kind of guilt? Definitely murder, abortion, giving a child away, some particularly unfair abandonment of a partner. If someone was guilty and did not want to look at his own fault, then his child, or even that child's child and perhaps the next child, may feel guilty. This deeply hidden guilt weakens the person internally and causes him to avoid certain areas and matters that could, based on associations, lead him to the trace of the past wrongdoing.

At one of the workshops, the representative of Derek's father started rubbing his hands intensively, as if he wanted to wash something off of them. The representative of the grandfather started making the same gesture. Some dramatic experience concerned him or someone from an even earlier generation. It was so hard that it was not assimilated mentally. The consequence was that the whole male line of the family became weakened. Derek could not take from his father, who was powerless and mentally half-absent, running away from any emotions and committing himself to work. Derek's father avoided emotionally charged topics so much that when I talked to him about his life for a while, without pressing him, he remained restless for some time later. As for Derek, he was timid and prone to compulsions, which usually indicate guilt.

So the unconscious sense of guilt and the resulting weakness are transmitted from one generation to another. However, this is not a transmission of some permanent pattern, because in each subsequent person, the "energy of guilt" manifests itself in a different way. The descendants experience not only guilt but also have unconscious knowledge about the event and the people involved (the latter is, of course, fully possible, since even strangers—representatives—access information about the details of other people's lives).

The Transgenerational Need for Balance

Already the previous subsection signaled an astonishing phenomenon—meddling of descendants in the affairs of their ancestors. It is more than just thinking about past events or judging them rationally. This phenomenon has a psychophysical and almost existential dimension of "being partly in the past." Sometimes it concerns someone from the family we knew or heard of, and sometimes it concerns a person we did not know and do not consciously think about at all.

Thirty-two-year-old Caroline called me for an appointment because, as she put it, she constantly met the "wrong men." In the constellation, she accused her grandfather of being "as he would be called today, a tyrant." In her opinion, this had a negative impact on three generations: Caroline's grandmother, aunt, and herself. The aunt, with whom the client felt connected, was reportedly particularly harmed. She had suffered from schizophrenia and had been in hospital for years. The constellation revealed that the grandfather was particularly bound to the dead, and his behavior was affected by his traumatic experiences. This was confirmed by Caroline's story—he fought against the Russians on the Eastern Front (he was a Silesian conscripted into the German army). The grandfather's sick daughter wanted to bear the hardships for him, even to be on the scene of the events that affected him, and she was also tied to those dead.

The client's task was to find respect for her grandfather and leave the past. It was very difficult for her, because she still needed to judge. She did not want to stop seeing her grandfather—perhaps quite aptly—as a tyrant. She even said that others had experienced the same he did, but behaved differently.

These words were a sign of loftiness. What happens when we judge so persistently? Mentally, we go against the current through generations, and we interfere in the affairs of our ancestors. This is more than a metaphor, this unconscious "activity" makes us internally involved. This is not without consequences for our psyche, as it is taking a great burden on ourselves. Caroline could not say: "I'm leaving it with respect." She could say: "I'm leaving it," but she could not add: "with respect." She still wanted to judge. The blind pursuit of imaginary justice was more important for her than her own well-being. Eventually, she managed to find respect for her grandfather and for what was connected with the war. Then she could leave the burden. There was also a representative in this constellation whom I referred to as the "man." Caroline felt that now she could look at him without fear, and the "man" also felt more attracted to her. The constellation showed that the client's attitude toward her grandfather shaped her relationships with men.[3]

In the above case, it was the person the client knew (grandfather) and also consciously thought about. She was only surprised by the strength with which she judged the grandfather. There are, however, situations where the client, during the constellation, is confronted with a previously completely unconscious need to bring about "justice." I remember constellations in which the clients began to feel a surprising desire for vengeance when the constellation revealed the perpetrators of some crime. This need for balance had already existed in them before, but they were not aware of its real object. In everyday life, it may have manifested itself in substitute forms, as entering into disputes and attempts to bring about "justice."

Catherine managed to start various ventures, but then she did not succeed and was constantly short of money. The business partners did not fulfill their obligations, the debtors did not pay their debts. The constellation showed that the probable killer (a member of the UPA[4]) of the grandmother's brother, was material here. Seeing that I manifested nervousness and mental tension in her grandmother's role, Catherine said that although outwardly the grandmother was very calm, she always felt her tension. However, when she shared her observations with her family, everyone opposed.

Catherine could not look at the perpetrator. But she could not look at her grandmother's brother either. She realized that she could not forgive the perpetrator, because it would be unfair on her grandmother. She sensed her anger (was it only anger at the perpetrator or also at the brother for risking his life?). In this way, she nursed her grandmother's sense of injustice, grudge against the brother, and partly her desire for revenge.

In her everyday life, Catherine did not think about the murder of her grandmother's brother and she did not want revenge. She became aware of her hidden feelings for those people and events only during the constellation. However, being in the grip of unconscious loyalty, judgment, and a transgenerational sense of grievance, she lost sight of what was right in business relations. She did not know whether she could demand outstanding money, expect proper payment. There had to be perpetrators and victims and a constant imbalance. This was due to the way she unconsciously experienced the events of her family's past.

PERINATAL DYNAMICS

Perinatal Acceptance of Life

A lot of people do not know how their birth went. And they usually do not care about this fact, not linking the circumstances of the birth to the events of their present life. And yet it has been known for a long time that the birth is an important event shaping man's psyche. Traditional cultures knew this well. Don C. Talayesva, an Indian from the Hopi tribe, talks about the circumstances of his birth (Talayesva 2013, 26 et seq.). He mentions the condition of the mother before the birth, the course of her pregnancy, the mother's superstitions connected with the pregnancy and, above all, the background of the birth, the actions taken at that time, the people involved or present in one way or another, he says who came, who left, what they said. Who of the members of our western culture could give an equally comprehensive description of their own births?

Systemic constellations prove the meaning of perinatal events, the traces of which remain in the mind of the individual and can be strong determinants of his behavior and fate. Caesarean section, the umbilical cord wrapped around him, prematurity and being in an incubator, as well as other events are the source of unconscious memories that affect functioning during his adulthood.

In constellations, we see not only what is confirmed by academic science, that is, the fact that the mental state of the mother during pregnancy and labor affects the development of the child's nervous system. They lead us to more extensive causal relationships. We can see that it is not only the influence of the current situation that is important, but also the circumstances of the birth of the woman who is now giving birth herself. These circumstances, if particularly difficult, may have left a mark on the child's psyche and shaped her relationship with the mother. When the child, already as an adult woman, gives birth to her own child, those events are in a way evoked and activated. Thus the child that is being born has to cope not only with the situation of his own birth, but often takes on himself the mother's mental states (or rather her inner child).

A difficult birth may result in a mentally "incomplete birth." It is like leaving part of oneself outside of oneself. It can also be described as a difficulty in accepting one's life, or a primary incomplete acceptance of life. An example is the situation of Violetta, who was apprehensive about her future. She saw her husband as unreliable, and finances and household matters were on her shoulders. She did not feel satisfaction in life. Her birth was difficult, she was wrapped by the umbilical cord. I positioned her and "life" and asked if she saw it, if she could look at it. She said it was like behind a curtain, there was some obstacle between her and "life." I set up this "obstacle"—the "obstacle" crouched in front of "life." When Violetta looked at the "obstacle," her mother came to her mind. Then she approached the "obstacle" and sat down next to it. She said she wanted the "obstacle" not to tremble, she wanted to help it. The "obstacle" said, however, that it was part of Violetta. I followed that feeling of the representative and told the client to take it as it was, that she did not need to change anything. Violetta put her head on the knees of the "obstacle," saying that she felt comfortable that she did not have to do anything. Later, Violetta asked if "life" "wanted her." I added her "birth" next to "life," then the "obstacle" withdrew. At the end, Violetta and the representatives of "life" and "birth" embraced each other. The client felt more complete. The obstacle was probably something heavy related to her birth, which Violetta rejected. Later, she approached it, "took it in," connected with it. She no longer ran away from that part of herself and her history. That is why she felt more complete.[5]

Accepting one's birth, life, and mother are processes that intertwine and cannot be treated as fully separate. Accepting one's birth is accepting the whole of oneself, including the neonatal "part," which, having experienced the trauma of birth, could have split off. Accepting one's life is connected with this.

Many people whose lives were endangered during or shortly after their birth remain as if in a "transition phase" between life and nonlife. They did not let themselves say, "It's over. I made it. I live like any other born man." This is naturally a hidden process and those people are not aware of it.

This state of affairs may have been due to the reactions of their environment. The parents and the family deeply experience the perinatal problems, and the child feels their emotions. It happens that once the child is born, the parents are not sure for some time whether he will survive. When it turns out that the child will live, there is no "ceremony of welcoming the child into the circle of the living." That is why the child may partially remain in the family's original emotions of life-threatening danger and never have enough strength to say to himself, "I'm alive!."

Paul's problem was frequent anxiety, diffidence, and emotional blockade in relations with women. He was born by caesarean section. I started the constellation by putting his representative on the side, saying he was a newborn, and chose a representative for his mother. The mother could not take care of the baby, she lay down on the floor. It was clear that she was like a baby herself. The constellation showed that she could not accept her parents as parents, she resisted strongly. This was probably influenced by the death of her father, who had died during the war when she had been six years old, and her mother's mourning, or maybe depression. But something else mattered here too. As Paul said, her mother "was given a random name, because she was thought to die." These words matched the constellation—Paul's mother did not take her life. Since "she was thought to die," she was not really alive even though she did survive. Paul added that every time his mother hugged him, he felt "some kind of theatre" in it. It was self-evident—because she did not take her own life, she could not show real affection.

Another important element was the caesarean section. The mother felt guilty about it; she felt that she did something wrong; she did not rise to the challenge. This is common in mothers in such situations—they feel insufficiently competent, incomplete, because the delivery required special intervention of doctors. However, since the mother is not satisfied with the childbirth, since it was not good or complete, the child cannot consider it complete, and thus cannot consider his life as fully valuable and take it as it is. He is alive, but not yet fully born.

As one can see, Paul's problem had at least two causes. One was the perinatal events that affected him, and the other was his mother's internal attitude, deeply rooted in the past. Probably, the latter was more crucial. Systemic constellations show that the strongest influence on the formation of the psyche comes from a relationship or from another psyche, and not from external events, in the strictly material sense.

Robert felt as if he had owed something to others all the time. And since he worked as a salesman, it was not inconsequential. He was constantly distracted, unable to save any money, and had the feeling that he wanted to lose everything. A constellation revealed the issue of an unknown, perhaps twin, sibling, as well as the father's earlier relationship and the client's loyalty to the mother. All these elements harmonized with the problem of feeling guilty, indebted.

Robert, however, felt again and again that "something was still unsettled." I took a piece of paper, put it on the floor, and said it was "what was still unresolved." We stood for a moment over the sheet, then the client said, "This is something simple." I stood on the piece of paper and immediately approached him with a smile and hugged him. There was something simple in it, and I was probably not a person, but some aspect of his life. Robert said that it was something "sunny" and that the words "I made it!" came to his mind. Something similar came to my mind too: "It's the end and the beginning at the same time." I realized that it was about the birth—about accepting the fact of birth, that it was successful, that it was all right. It was not until later that I remembered Robert telling me that before his birth, his father was so scared that he did not come home. His mother was also scared.

The Unknown Twin

Real-life examples show that the bond between twin siblings is particularly strong. Researchers of monozygotic twins noticed that those who were separated in childhood are even more alike in terms of personality traits, habits, and lifelines than those that were reared together (Dossey 2013). Perhaps separated twins, often unaware of one another's existence, stick together more closely. After all, in constellations, we observe that it is the lack of knowledge and access to a loved one that strengthens identification with him. Thanks to constellations, we also know how strong the influence of a twin sibling is if he dies before he is born. There are many more twin pregnancies, than born twins; so it is not uncommon to know nothing about the existence of the twin. Lawrence Wright, expressing the importance of this fact, writes:

> Although only about one out of eighty or ninety live births produces twins, at least one-eighth of all natural pregnancies begin as twins. Many of us singletons, in other words, began life as something more—as part of a pair. (Wright 1995, 52)

Karen wanted to work on her relationship. During her constellation—which is not surprising—her attitude toward the parents came to light. However, when we worked through this issue to some extent, Karen still felt anxious, which prevented me from completing the constellation. In such a case, when a lot has already been done and the client still does not feel satisfied, I put a piece of paper in front of him as "something that also matters here" or "something that causes this anxiety." That is what I did this time too.

I stood on the piece of paper and followed the intuitive movement. I crouched and looked down. Karen clearly felt that she was bound to the person I represented. Some unusual sense of superiority arose in her, she wanted to "take in, absorb" this person, and a moment later, those triumphant and aggressive—as I would call them—feelings turned into love. I felt an impulse to stand up. I stood next to the client. She finally felt good. She said it was as if her late husband, who had come to life, was standing next to her. However, Karen was never married. I found it was rather reminiscent of a different situation. As usual in such cases, I noted that these were only assumptions and associations, and said it could be her dead twin. At this point, the client moved and said that when she was 16, she had a cyst removed. The doctor then said that it was her twin that had been absorbed by her during the fetal period. Interestingly, she unconsciously used the word "absorbed" when she described her attitude toward the unknown person in the constellation.

Joanna, a young woman, felt insecure both in her relationship with her partner and at work. She had the feeling that it would "come out," that she "did not qualify," that she was "out of place," and that she was "cheating" (so she manifested symptoms of the phenomenon that has its own name—impostor syndrome). She said that she often had some involuntary fantasies that depicted her condition. In one of these fantasies, someone tore her asymmetrically into two parts; in another one, someone ripped her skin off, scraping her body on the pavement, first one side, then the other; in yet another one, someone crushed her with a flagstone.

The conversation showed that she felt something like her *alter ego*, an "inner saboteur" or something of that kind. I asked her to name that part of herself and write the name down on a piece of paper. The client wrote: "Her." She put the sheet on the floor, and I stood on it as a representative. The client felt that I came to “punish” her, but I had no negative attitude toward her. Nevertheless, there was something strange between us that I could not fully define. As if I had a vague feeling that there had been or still was some kind of dispute or rivalry between us. At one point, I sat in the armchair that the client had previously occupied and felt good in it.

In the further part of the constellation, I wondered what sentences of strength would be the solution. We both agreed that they would be: “You’re here too” and “Take part in what I do.” All this gave the impression of both rivalry as well as bond and identification. This is the case for twins.

The existence of the unknown, dead twin causes many repercussions in the survivor’s emotional life. It often results in an unexplained longing that most people project onto their relationships, which makes them unsuccessful.

A certain syndrome of emotions and behaviors is characteristic. It involves an irrational sense of guilt, sometimes an emotional oscillation between aggressiveness and timidity, between demanding and submissiveness is also characteristic. This aggregate of feelings refers to the events that took place in the womb, where the bond and love and rivalry between the twins intertwined. When one of them was dying, there was a feeling of guilt about surviving and striving for life. It seems that many single twins in adulthood experience strong feelings of rivalry yet they are unable to take any action to achieve what they reportedly want. Additionally, they feel extremely lonely.

Patrick constantly “felt inferior,” he was quiet and avoided rivalry. At the same time, he was overwhelmed by enormous jealousy that paralyzed his actions completely. It was first of all directed at his cousin. During our many meetings, he constantly drew a polarized picture: him—quiet, always concerned about what others feel and forgetting about himself, and his cousin—selfish, smiling, and doing better. Him—constantly criticized, his cousin—given as an example (although in fact the cousin did not achieve much). When he found out about any of his cousin’s moves in life, it was as if all the energy left him. It was as if he was connected to his cousin or played a continuous zero-sum game with him—whenever his cousin gained something, whether a good word or a new drill, Patrick felt as if he lost it. It looked as if all the manifestations of his cousin’s life, even the fact that he lived somewhere, took Patrick’s life away.

Also, Patrick was not able to distance himself from the opinion of his environment—he kept asking what others thought about this or that. He could not choose anything by himself, constantly looking for a confirmation of his choices in his environment. When, for instance, he wanted to buy a bicycle, he asked everyone what kind of bike they thought he should buy; they suggested different ones, and finally he did not buy any. As if he had lived "outside," and not his life. He looked around all the time. As a child, he had a great need for praise, but he dread that he had done something wrong and that someone would be angry with him. And he wanted to avoid this so much that he avoided any kind of activity. What was the pattern here? Patrick behaved like a man on release after a long sentence—he felt that everyone looked at him, judged him, generally had a bad opinion of him, and he constantly had to beware.

The above states were not trivial. Although Patrick reflected on what was happening to him, he could not in any way stop his feelings, and these paralyzed his life and development completely.

Of course, the cousin was not the point. Because they knew each other since childhood, and certain facts—such as comparing the two boys—matched Patrick's emotions, the cousin became a perfect substitute for someone else.

The constellation showed that Patrick was tied to someone completely unknown to him. After the constellation, many workshop participants, even though they knew nothing about Patrick, said that they associated this unknown person with his twin.

SYSTEMIC-PSYCHODYNAMIC TRANSDUCTION

By eliminating negative influences of the system, constellations in a way purify our psyche and enable it to function better. Not always, however, everything that is problematic disappears after a constellation. Where can the problem still be, since it is no longer in the system? Of course, in our individually understood mind, in our personality, and in our character.

I believe that systemic influences press on the psyche and unconsciously shape our personality from the prenatal period. They are one of the elements that, next to ordinary perception, thoughts, traumas, fantasies, or emotions, constitute the building blocks of our personality. In other words, from an early age, without being aware of it, we live with the thought that our father was missing his father, that the grandmother's child was harmed, that we would like to change our grandfather's tragic life, that our older siblings were aborted, or that we have a departed twin, and so on. These often dramatic histories, hard experiences, and interrupted bonds are what shapes our mind, character, and its problematic spheres daily.

I refer to this process as systemic-psychodynamic transduction. As a result of this process, the systemic influence creates a more or less permanent "record" in our psyche. That is why when we change the character of this impact from negative to positive during a constellation, not everything is changed. This situation can be compared to an event when a stone falls into the wheels of a machine and slowly damages them during its operation. After the stone is removed, the machine may still work incorrectly, as the permanently damaged parts behave as when the stone was stuck in them. This is the case, for example, in schizophrenia, autism, or other severe disorders, for the treatment of which systemic constellations alone are often not enough, although they are sometimes very important in this process.

Such mental states as those referred to as borderline personality disorder, or at least some of them, would be determined by unconscious knowledge of the existence of a twin sibling who died in the womb. Because the systemic impact is permanent, having a deceased twin is like being accompanied by him and at the same time constant re-experiencing of the past conflict with him. This may account for the characteristic oscillations between idealization and devaluation, as well as for mood lability.

Narcissism, on the other hand, that we can understand as an attempt to identify with a created image, may result from entanglement with someone with whom the subject unconsciously identifies himself. Alienation from oneself would cause a compulsion to create a "substitute" identity (Janus 2019, 109 et seq.). Of course, the factors mentioned would not be the only ones that shape the above disorders, but they would be some of the most important ones.

Also less serious psychological problems may result from the permanent shaping of the psyche by systemic influence. During psychoanalytic therapy Matthew told me that he often had thoughts and dreams in which it turned out that he was "cheated by the matrix," as he figuratively put it. He imagined that "they would find out that he was inferior, that he was a subhuman, some sort of freak." He described it metaphorically: "It's as if it turned out that I don't have a dick when I'm in the cloakroom with basketball players," "I don't have arms, legs," "I have some fundamental deficit on the biological level." He happened to take narcotics, from which he remembered impressions as if "demons created that whole day, that situation." He also had dreams, when he barely fell asleep, in which someone attacked him.

Matthew had a specific family situation. He had older siblings, and his father often stayed away from home, where his mother's friend was hosted for years and took care of him. Because something bothered him, he took genetic tests around the age of thirty. It turned out that his biological father was that man, the mother's friend. Both the mother and his biological father claimed that they knew nothing about it. His fears and fantasies could be understood as the expression of unconscious perception of his true family system. Matthew "knew" that someone else was his father and that his official family was a kind of "matrix." He felt that something could "come out," he also felt a "fundamental deficit" and that he was "inferior." In this way, Matthew's psyche was shaped over the years by the perception that only took place on the unconscious level. This perception modified his attitude to his mother, to his father, to his mother's friend, and to his siblings. It influenced the shape of his Oedipus complex. All these factors formed his personality.

If this process really exists, our understanding of mental development and the factors that influence it should be radically transformed. It probably plays a role in each of us, cocreating our character. It could also explain the frequent cases in which we have no idea how these and no other traits may have developed in a given individual. An example is psychopathy that developed in a person who was brought up with care. Perhaps one becomes a psychopath neither because of his genes nor as a result of his upbringing, but through the systemic factors that had an impact on him when he was a child. In other words, the parents may have been caring, and there were no traumas in the child's life, but his psyche "stayed" in a very unfavorable, perhaps somewhat traumatic environment (transgenerational losses, abandonments, secrets, maybe crimes). Such a situation may have led to the development of certain defense mechanisms, for example, suppression of emotionality and empathy, and development of a specific attitude to the world.

NOTES

1. The genocide of Poles carried out by Ukrainian nationalists, with the support of the Ukrainian citizens, in the prewar territories of Poland (now Ukraine) in 1943–1945. During the slaughter, Ukrainians killed over 50,000 people, mostly whole families, in a sadistic way.

2. Józef Klemens Piłsudski, politician and soldier, chief commander of the Polish Army (from November 1918), chief of state (1918–1922), and first marshal of Poland. Considered to be the founder of Polish independence after the period of partitions, when Poland disappeared from the map of Europe (1795–1918). Piłsudski commanded the Polish army during the Polish-Bolshevik war of 1919–1921. This war was fought by reborn Poland against postrevolutionary Russia commanded by Lenin and the Bolshevik party. Russia's goal was to subjugate Poland and to transfer the revolution to Germany and Western Europe. Polish troops won the decisive battles, which caused that the Russians retreated and made peace possible.

3. One can also consider what cause and effect relationships were here. The initial interview showed that Caroline divided the world of men into the "well-behaved" but uninteresting ones, and those "with problems" and "burdened" that interested her, although they turned out to be a source of suffering. She read me a list of the qualities she wanted a man to have—but it was difficult to say whether she wanted to meet such a man or whether she wanted the "bad guys" to eventually become like that. Perhaps her dilemmas expressed an unconscious need to reconcile with her "bad" grandfather and end the female judgments in her family.

4. Ukrainian Insurgent Army (UPA)—an armed formation established in 1942 by Ukrainian nationalists. The aim of the UPA was to build independent Ukraine. During World War II, its members fought against the occupying German authorities, Russians, and Poles, whom they also regarded as occupiers. At certain times, the UPA cooperated with Nazi Germany against the Red Army, Soviet, and Polish partisans. It was also active in the first years after the war in the USSR and in the east of Poland. It

is coresponsible for the terrible massacre of Poles, the so-called Volhynian slaughter, during the German occupation of eastern Poland in 1943–1945.

5. After the constellation, the representative of the "obstacle" added: "I was alternately her male and her female part." Violetta's daughter is bisexual. Perhaps the daughter took on herself something that came from or through her mother and was related to gender.

Bibliography

Austermann Alfred, and Bettina Austermann. 2019. *Drama in the Womb: The Surviving Twin Syndrome*, translated by Gabriele Sick and Leni Rice. Berlin: Königsweg Verlag.

Breland, Keller, and Marian Breland. 1961. "The Misbehavior of Organisms." *American Psychologist*, 16: 681–684.

Brottman, Mikita. 2011. *Phantoms of the Clinic: From Thought-Transference to Projective Identification*. London: Karnac Books. Kindle.

Cannon, Mary, Peter B. Jones, and Robin M. Murray. 2002. "Obstetric complications and schizophrenia: Historical and meta-analytic review." *American Journal of Psychiatry*, 159(7): 1080–1092.

Carnabucci, Karen, and Ronald Anderson. 2012. *Integrating Psychodrama and Systemic Constellation Work: New Directions for Action Methods, Mind-Body Therapies and Energy Healing*. London, PA: Jessica Kingsley Publishers. Kindle.

Crowhurst, Brenton, and E. M. Coles. 1989. "Kurt Schneider's concepts of psychopathy and schizophrenia: A review of the English literature." *Canadian Journal of Psychiatry*, 34(3): 238–243.

Davies, Paul. 2019. *The Demon in the Machine: How Hidden Webs of Information Are Solving the Mystery of Life*. Chicago, IL: The University of Chicago Press.

Dossey, Larry. 2013. *One Mind: How Our Individual Mind is Part of a Greater Consciousness and Why it Matters*. New York City: Hay House.

Dreher, Henry. 1996. *The Immune Power Personality: Seven Traits You Can Develop to Stay Healthy*. London: Penguin Books.

Ehrenwald, Jan. 1947. *Telepathy and Medical Psychology*. London: George Allen & Unwin Ltd.

Eisenbud, Jule. 1952. "The Use of the Telepathy Hypothesis in Psychotherapy." In *Specialized Techniques in Psychotherapy*, edited by Gustav Bychowski and J. Louise Despert, pp. 41–63. New York: Grove Press.

Estés, Clarissa Pinkola. 2013. *Untie the Strong Woman: Blessed Mother's Immaculate Love for the Wild Soul*. Boulder, CO: Sounds True.

Ferenczi, Sándor. 1995. *The Clinical Diary of Sándor Ferenczi*, translated by Michael Balint and Nicola Zarday Jackson, edited by Judith Dupont. Cambridge, London: Harvard University Press.

Fink, Bruce. 1997. *A Clinical Introduction to Lacanian Psychoanalysis*. Cambridge, MA: Harvard University Press.

Franke, Ursula. 2003. *In My Mind's Eye: Family Constellations in Individual Therapy and Counselling*. Heidelberg: Carl-Auer-Systeme Verlag.

Freud, Sigmund. 1955. "A childhood recollection from *Dichtung und Wahrheit*." In *The Standard Edition of the Complete Psychological Works of Sigmund Freud*, translated and edited by James Strachey, vol. 17, pp. 145–156. London: Hogarth Press.

———. 1957. "Some character types met with in psychoanalytic work." In *The Standard Edition of the Complete psychological works of Sigmund Freud*, translated and edited by James Strachey, vol. 14, pp. 309–333. London: Hogarth Press.

———. 1990. *New Introductory Lectures on Psycho-Analysis*. New York: W.W. Norton & Company.

Greyson, Bruce. 1977. "Telepathy in mental illness: Deluge or delusion?" *The Journal of Nervous and Mental Disease*, 165(3): 184–200.

Grün, Anselm, and Friedrich Assländer. 2009. *Jak kierować ludźmi?*, translated by Małgorzata Witwicka. Kraków: Wydawnictwo Salwator.

Hausner, Stephan. 2011. *Even if it Costs Me My Life. Systemic Constellations and Serious Illness*. New York: Routledge.

Hellinger, Bert. 2001. *Love's Own Truths: Bonding and Balancing in Close Relationships*, translated by Maureen Oberli-Turner and Hunter Beaumont. Phoenix: Zeig, Tucker & Theisen.

———. 2003. *To the Heart of the Matter: Brief Therapies*, translated by Colleen Beaumont. Heidelberg: Carl-Auer-Systeme Verlag.

———. 2004. *Listy terapeutyczne. Znaleźć to, co działa*, translated by Zenon Mazurczak. Warszawa: Wydawnictwo Jacek Santorski & Co.

———. 2008. *Die Liebe des Geistes: Was zu ihr führt und wie sie gelingt*. Bischofswiesen: Hellinger Publications.

———. 2008a. *Glück, das bleibt: Wie Beziehungen gelingen*. Stuttgart: Verlag Kreuz.

———. 2008b. *Porządki pomagania. Czyli jak, kiedy i komu skutecznie pomagać*. Warszawa: Wydawnictwo Jacek Santorski & Co.

———. 2011. *Laws of Healing: Getting Well, Staying Well*, translated by Angelika Schenk, edited by Suzi Tucker. Bischofswiesen: Hellinger Publications.

———. 2011a. *Erfolge im Leben und im Beruf*. Bischofswiesen: Hellinger Publications.

———. 2014. *Nowa świadomość. Duchowy wymiar ustawień rodzin*, translated by Katarzyna Preiss-Jastrzębska. Warszawa: Wydawnictwo Czarna Owca.

———. 2014a. *Neue Geschichten: Zwei*. Bischofswiesen: Hellinger Publications.

———. 2014b. *Neue Geschichten: Drei*. Bischofswiesen: Hellinger Publications.

———. 2016. *Nowe rozważania 1. Wiedzieć skąd*, translated by Katarzyna Preiss-Jastrzębska. Warszawa: Wydawnictwo Virgo.

Hellinger, Bert, and Hanne-Lore Heilmann. 2018. *Mein Leben. Mein Werk.* München: Ariston Verlag.
Hellinger, Bert, and Gabriele ten Hövel. 1999. *Acknowledging What Is: Conversations with Bert Hellinger*, translated by Colleen Beaumont. Phoenix, Arizona: Zeig, Tucker & Co., Inc.
Hellinger, Bert, and Andrzej Nehrebecki. 2012. *Miłość zaklęta w chorobie.* Kraków: Wydawnictwo Pocieszka.
Hellinger, Bert, and Gerhard Walper. n.d. "Bert Hellinger zur Weiterentwicklung seiner Arbeit und zu seinen Erfahrungen mit Autismus: Ein Interview von Gerhard Walper." Accessed March 2, 2019. https://www.hellinger.com/index.php?id=100.
Henle, Mary. 1986. *1879 and All That: Essays in the Theory and History of Psychology.* New York: Columbia University Press.
ICD-10 Version: 2019. n.d. "Chapter V: Mental and behavioural disorders, (F00-F99)." Accessed March 9, 2021. https://icd.who.int/browse10/2019/en#/F20-F29.
Janus, Damian. 2019. *Psychopathology and Religion: Structural Convergences between Mental Disorders and Religion*, translated by Barbara Gąstoł. Lanham, Boulder, New York, London: Lexington Books.
Kamińska, Anna. 2016. *Odnalezieni. Prawdziwe historie adoptowanych.* Kraków: Wydawnictwo Literackie.
Kampenhout, Daan van. 2006. *Rytuały szamańskie a ustawienia rodzinne*, translated by Małgorzata Baworowska. Katowice: Wydawnictwo KOS.
Karpowicz, Paweł. 2007. "Droga szczęśliwego dziecka." *ALBO albo. Problemy psychologii i kultury*, no. 1 (43). Warszawa: ENETEIA.
Kets de Vries, Manfred F. R. 2006. *The Leader on the Couch: A Clinical Approach to Changing People and Organizations.* San Francisco, CA: Jossey-Bass.
Lacan, Jacques. 1938. *Family Complexes in the Formation of the Individual*, translated by Cormac Gallagher. Chippenham: Antony Rowe Ltd.
Laing, R. D., and Aaron Esterson. 2017. *Sanity, Madness and the Family: Families of Schizophrenics.* London, New York: Routledge.
LeShan, Lawrence. 1994. *Cancer as a Turning Point: A Handbook for People with Cancer, Their Families, and Health Professionals.* Middlesex: Penguin Books.
Lowen, Alexander. 1974. *Depression and The Body: The Biological Basis of Faith and Reality.* Baltimore, MA: Penguin Books.
———. 2004. *Love, Sex and Your Heart.* Alachua, FL: Bioenergetics Press.
Manné, Joy. 2013. *Conceptual Constellations: Constellating Story and Archetype.* CreateSpace. Kindle.
Moreno, Jacob Levy, and Zerka T. Moreno. 2011. *Psychodrama, Second Volume: Foundations of Psychotherapy.* U.K.: The North-West Psychodrama Association.
Musser, George. 2015. *Spooky Action at a Distance. The Phenomenon That Reimagines Space and Time-and What It Means for Black Holes, the Big Bang, and Theories of Everything.* New York: Scientific American/Farrar, Straus and Giroux.
Osiński, Włodzimierz Adam. 2017. *Czwarty Wymiar*, March (3).
Prekop, Jirina. 2015. *Rodzina żyje miłością. Jak odbudować zdrowe i głębokie więzi*, translated by Anna Choińska. Warszawa: Wydawnictwo Czarna Owca.

Quinodoz, Jean-Michel. 2008. *Listening to Hanna Segal: Her Contribution to Psychoanalysis*, translated by David Alcorn, edited by Dana Birksted-Breen. London, New York: Routledge.

Rogers, Jenny. 2012. *Coaching Skills: A Handbook*. Maidenhead: Open University Press.

Røine, Eva. 1997. *Psychodrama: Group Psychotherapy as Experimental Theatre: Playing the Leading Role in Your Own Life*, translated by Ann Zwik. London and Bristol, PA: Jessica Kingsley Publishers.

Ruppert, Franz. 2012. *Symbiosis and Autonomy: Symbiotic Trauma and Love Beyond Entanglements*, translated by Julia Stuebs and Rick Hosburn, edited by Vivian Broughton. Steyning: Green Balloon Publishing.

Ruppert, Franz, Birgit Assel, Doris Brombach, Vivian Broughton, Annemarie Denk, Christina Freund, Gabriele Hoppe, et al. 2016. *Early Trauma: Pregnancy, Birth and First Years of Life*, translated by Julia Stuebs and Rick Hosburn, edited by Vivian Broughton. Steyning: Green Balloon Publishing.

Samuels, Andrew, Bani Shorter, and Fred Plaut. 2013. *A Critical Dictionary of Jungian Analysis*. Hove, New York: Routledge.

Shafer, Matthew, and Daniela Schiller. 2020. "The Brain's social road maps." *Scientific American*, 322(2): 30–35.

Schober-Howorka, Jasmin. 2012. *Family Constellation and Past Lives*. Lulu.com.

Simon, Richard. 1992. *One on One: Conversations with the Shapers of Family Therapy*. New York, London: The Guilford Press.

Simonton, Oscar Carl. 2004. "Hope and the Healing Journey." Filmed March 13 at The Simonton Cancer Center and Visiting Nurse & Hospice Care, Santa Barbara, CA. Video. http://www.ahealth.com/content/education/media/.

Simonton, Oscar Carl, Stephanie Matthews-Simonton, and James Creighton. 1978. *Getting Well Again: A Step-By-Step Self-Help Guide to Overcoming Cancer for Patients and Their Families*. Los Angeles: J.P. Tarcher.

Simonton, Oscar Carl, Reid M. Henson, and Brenda Hampton. 1992. *The Healing Journey*. New York, Toronto, London, Sydney, Auckland: Bantam Books.

Soares, Christine. 2009. "Primal programs." *Scientific American*, 300(5): 17–18.

Schreber, Daniel Paul. 2000. *Memoirs of My Nervous Illness*, translated and edited by Ida Macalpine and Richard A. Hunter. New York: New York Review Books Classics.

Słodkowski, Jędrzej. 2014. *Jestem hetero. Nie jestem mężczyzną, który po prostu się przebiera. Tu chodzi o coś więcej*. Published September 20, 2014. http://www.wysokieobcasy.pl/wysokie-obcasy/1,96856,16655417, Jestem_hetero__Nie_jestem_mezczyzna__ktory_po_prostu.html.

Sparrer, Insa. 2006. *Systemische Strukturaufstellungen: Theorie und Praxis*. Heidelberg: Carl Auer Systeme.

Talarczyk, Małgorzata. 2011. "Family constellation method of Bert Hellinger in the context of the Code of Ethics for Psychotherapists." *Archives of Psychiatry and Psychotherapy*, 3: 65–74. Kraków: Polskie Towarzystwo Psychiatryczne.

Talayesva, Don C. 2013. *Sun Chief: The Autobiography of a Hopi Indian*, edited by Leo W. Simmons. New Haven: Yale University Press.

Temoshok, Lydia, and Henry Dreher. 1992. *The Type C Connection: The Behavioral Links to Cancer and Your Health*. New York: Random House.

Ulsamer, Bertold. 1999. *Ohne Wurzeln keine Flügel. Die systemische Therapie von Bert Hellinger*. München: Goldmann.

———. 2001. *Das Handwerk des Familien-Stellens. Eine Einführung In die Praxis der systemischen Hellinger-Therapie*. München: Arkana.

Varga von Kibéd, Matthias, and Insa Sparrer. 2018. *Ganz im Gegenteil: Tetralemmaarbeit und andere Grundformen Systemischer Strukturaufstellungen—für Querdenker, und solche die es werden wollen*. Heidelberg: Carl-Auer Systeme Verlag.

Watkins, John. 2008. *Hearing Voices: A Common Human Experience*. Melbourne: Michelle Anderson Publishing.

Whittington, John. 2016. *Systemic Coaching and Constellations: The Principles, Practices and Applications for Individuals, Teams and Groups*. London, PA, New Delhi: Kogan Page.

Wirga, Mariusz. 1998. *Zwyciężyć chorobę*. Katowice: Wydawnictwo KOS.

Wolynn, Mark. 2016. *It Didn't Start with You: How Inherited Family Trauma Shapes Who We Are and How to End the Cycle*. New York: Viking.

Wright, Lawrence. 1995. "A Reporter at large: Double mystery." *New Yorker*, 7: 45–62.

Zdrada, Damian. 2017. *Seksoholizm. Perwersja i miłość*. Warszawa: Difin.

Index

About the Author

Damian Janus graduated from the faculties of psychology, philosophy, and religious studies at the Jagiellonian University (Krakow, Poland) and has specializations in clinical psychology and psycho-oncology. He participated in training courses in Gestalt psychotherapy, bodywork, psychodynamic psychotherapy, and Lacanian psychoanalysis. He completed trainings in family constellations and new family constellations. He worked in a psychiatric ward, mental health clinic, addiction treatment clinic, and has a private psychotherapeutic practice. He is interested in physics and the history of science and technology.

www.ingramcontent.com/pod-product-compliance
Lightning Source LLC
LaVergne TN
LVHW091533200926
848483LV00002B/388